THE
PRINCIPLES AND ART
OF
CURE BY HOMOEOPATHY

The Principles and Art of Cure by Homœopathy

A MODERN TEXTBOOK

BY

HERBERT A. ROBERTS, M.D.

Chairman, American Foundation for Homœopathy;
Head of Department of Homœopathic Philosophy,
Postgraduate School of the American Foundation;
Ex-President, International Hahnemannian Association;
Editor, *Homœopathic Recorder*; Author of the *Principles and
Practicability of Bœnninghausen's Therapeutic Pocket Book*;
Sensations As If——; *The Rheumatic Remedies*; *The Study of
Remedies by Comparison*

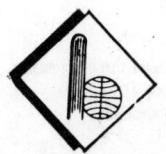

B. Jain Publishers Pvt. Ltd.
USA — EUROPE — INDIA

THE PRINCIPLES AND ART OF CURE BY HOMOEOPATHY

Low Price Edition: 2002
17th Impression: 2016

Published by Kuldeep Jain for
B. JAIN PUBLISHERS (P) LTD.
1921/10, Chuna Mandi, Paharganj, New Delhi 110 055 (INDIA)
Tel.: +91-11-4567 1000   Fax: +91-11-4567 1010
Email: info@bjain.com   Website: www.bjain.com

Printed in India by
B.B Press, Noida

ISBN: 978-81-319-0148-9

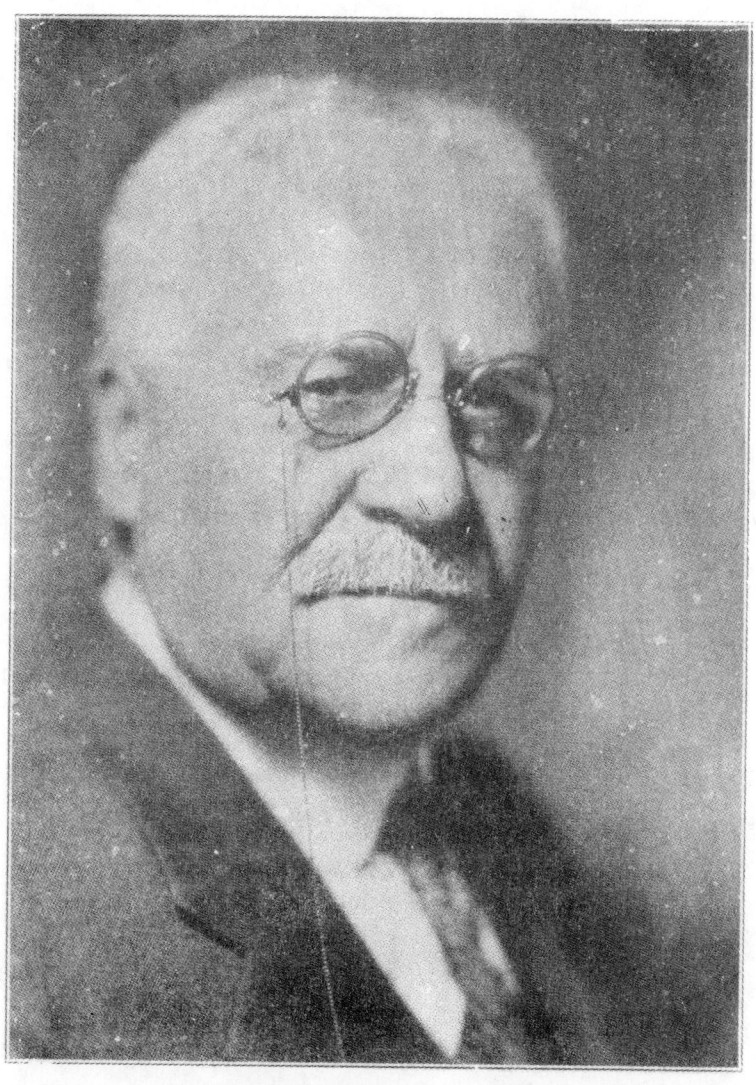

HERBERT A. ROBERTS, M.D.
Chairman Board of Editors, The Homoeopathic Recorder
1928-1937

THIS WORK IS DEDICATED
TO ALL SEEKERS AFTER TRUTH IN HEALING
OF EVERY AGE AND RACE

PREFACE

THE first question asked of us who profess to uphold Hahnemann's teaching is this : What is Homœopathy ? Why is Homœopathy preferable to other methods of medical practice ?

How shall we answer it ? Is it true that we can answer it by saying : Homœopathy is a system of medicine ? The thoughtful, conscientious homœopathic physician will feel that a more comprehensive answer must be given, an answer that will appeal to the sense of logic in the mind of the questioner.

We believe that Homœopathy has no standing if it cannot be definitely proven that it stands firmly upon the basis of fundamental natural laws. In this book the author has tried to show the " logical reasonableness of homœopathy ", as Carroll Dunham termed it.

Here an attempt has been made to correlate the principles that govern the homœopathic methods of healing with those principles and laws that govern all life : i.e. motion, growth, development. No one realizes more than the author that these efforts are imperfect and incomplete, but if they serve to inspire further research along the lines of the fundamental oneness of Homœopathy with Universal Law, his object will have been attained.

To Sir J. C. Bose, R. A. Millikan, A. H. Compton and others, the author is indebted for the use of material, the fruit of their labours.

In one group of chapters, the student of homœopathic philosophy will note that few original thoughts have been incorporated ; he will be able to trace the source of many of these thoughts, and even paragraphs, to Hahnemannian students who have put into clear, concise phrases the teaching that best reaches the novice, and that appeals to the seasoned homœopathician as the best testimony that could be offered. Many of the choicest bits of homœopathic philosophy are scattered through homœopathic literature, and it is to gather

• these into compact form, and so place the best thought upon homœopathic philosophy in accessible place for student and physician alike, that this work has been attempted.

The author of this book has spent many fruitful hours in searching the printed records left by many stalwarts in the homœopathic vanguard, and not only have the printed works of individual authors been closely scanned for the material found here, but old volumes of homœopathic magazines long since out of print have yielded valuable material.

It has been our experience of several years that when the principles of Hahnemannian homœopathy have been set before the student in a manner that appeals to his sense of logic, he readily grasps it and is able to incorporate it into practical application. It has been our aim in this book so to set forth the principles underlying the practice of Hahnemannian homœopathy that they could be grasped and made of practical application in the healing art.

To Hahnemann, Bœnninghausen, Hering, Joslin, Lippe, Fincke, Carroll Dunham, P. P. Wells, A. R. Morgan, T. F. Allen, H. C. Allen, J. H. Allen, James Tyler Kent, Stuart Close, C. M. Boger, and others ; and to the members of the International Hahnemannian Association, who by precept and example have stimulated thought, the author is deeply indebted for the source of material. If any profit from this book, let him remember the hosts of people healed by these physicians who staked their whole method of practice on the fundamental laws of healing, and be encouraged thereby in the knowledge that to him also is the same power, and in exactly the same degree in which he employs these fundamental laws.

H. A. ROBERTS.

Derby, Conn.
January 10th, 1936.

PREFACE TO THE SECOND EDITION

OUT of the strain and stress and havoc and horror of this present world conflict comes the call for a new edition of this book. The remainder of the former edition having been destroyed during the attacks on London, this call for a new edition is a small part of the answer of the democracies to the attempt to enslave and dominate all free peoples. It epitomizes the struggle to perpetuate the ideals for which the democracies stand—the opportunity to develop and express individuality in every way consonant with the good of the whole.

We believe that in the course of time and by the action of natural laws, the world will be cured of its present evils and will go on to greater health of all its parts.

Natural law is immutable. We judge by finite measurements, but our convictions relate our finite perspective to ultimate—and infinite—acceptance of these laws, which will right the equilibrium in the individual, the nation, and the world.

This edition is more than a reprint ; chapters of importance have been added particularly on the endocrine glands, on the release of atomic energy by potentization, and some dangers in modern medication ; but few changes have been made in the original chapters of the text.

H. A. ROBERTS.

Derby, Conn.
1942.

CONTENTS

CHAPTER I

WHAT HAS HOMŒOPATHY TO OFFER THE YOUNG MAN?

WHAT has homœopathy to offer the young man as a future? This question comes to us repeatedly and in our changing economic conditions it is a pertinent question.

Perhaps we can get at the problem best by asking the young man the counter-question: " What do you want to get out of life? " Only his honest reply to the question can throw any light upon his adaptability to homœopathy and only upon an honest consideration of his adaptability can we prophesy what homœopathy has to offer him. Why is he thinking of studying medicine?

Is he lazy and does he consider a profession an easy way to earn a living? Does he look upon medicine as a profession to be sought because of its honourable place in the community or as a position to be desired to secure a standing in society? Has he an ambition to be hailed as a great surgeon or bacteriologist? Is he thinking first of the possible financial returns?

If he would use his foothold as a physician for a life of ease, for a position in the community or in society, or for a means of obtaining fame or wealth, homœopathy offers him little that he would care to accept.

How does he react to the fads of the day, the bulletins of the laboratories, the specious advertising of pharmaceutical houses, the glib talk of salesmen? Does he believe that colloids are, after all, homœopathic potentiations? Or is he convinced that colloidal preparations are but recent and crude imitations of homœopathic potentiation which are inferior and far more uncertain in their effects than the proven homœopathic remedy?

If he replies to your question of his idea of the direction of his future so that it leads you to think that he looks upon sick humanity as suffering men and women, that he has a burning

13

desire to serve them, to help them to better health and therefore greater usefulness and happiness, then you may be sure there is a sound foundation upon which he may build a plan of life in which homœopathy will offer him great reward. We can proceed further with our probing of his character and abilities, and determine what homœopathy has to offer him by finding out what he has to offer homœopathy.

One of the first essentials, now that we are convinced of his unselfish desire to serve, is to determine whether he has stability. If he is mercurial in temperament, easily influenced, and finds it difficult to hold a straight course, always seeking the easiest way, do not encourage him to study homœopathy.

Homœopathy is founded upon principles that are in turn founded upon natural laws. If homœopathy is founded upon natural laws, it is as basic and eternal as the hills ; more, natural laws were formulated before the hills came into being. If a man follows where homœopathy leads, he must be able to follow those laws and to hold close to them regardless of the pressure of influence.

Stability of character must have with it, and in equal measure, the quality of patience. In ordinary medicine the quality of patience seemingly is not so necessary, since we too frequently find that in extreme cases where things have taken an undesirable course the physician comforts himself that " everything possible has been done for the patient ". In homœopathy, one of our greatest axioms is : WHEN IN DOUBT, DON'T. The homœopathic physician must be able to plan his course, and once having determined upon it, to stick to it until he finds good reason for changing his course ; he must be able to wait.

The man who considers homœopathy as a possible future must be a student of people and willing to become a student of philosophy. He must be able to read between the true and the false in any symptoms the patient may give ; he must possess a sense of values. He must train himself to observe all those signs which the vital energy writes upon the human face, and he must be able to interpret all the signs, which show through habits and circumstances, into indications for the health-restoring medicines which he has at his command. Hours must be spent in patient study, tracing the course of the disturbance and the remedy to fit it, always basing the process upon the sound rock of natural law.

To the young man who is equipped, and willing to undergo the training for this lifelong task, homœopathy has everything to offer.

In the first place, homœopathy offers to the independent mind an opportunity continually to seek new verifications of the natural laws upon which this system of medicine is based. It opens up vast fields to the pioneer, and we cannot gauge the distance that eager minds may travel, nor how greatly the interpretations of these laws may influence the civilization of the future.

Homœopathy offers a life of service to humanity, and it is the only method of healing that surely sets the sick man and sick woman on the permanent road to recovery. We must remember that though we may fail, the failure is ours ; it is not the failure of homœopathy. The better knowledge we have of the " tools of our trade " the better use we should make of them.

Homœopathy treats the sick individual ; it is therefore a specialty. In spite of the trend toward group practice, group thinking and even group mode of life as seen all about us to-day, we have yet to be convinced that the man is not greater than the mass and that as long as intelligent thinking people realize and prize their individuality, the individual approach will hold an appeal to them. Therefore, homœo-pathy offers a special inducement to the man who can teach people to think and act as individuals, and to demand medical treatment as individuals.

Homœopathy considers the man as a whole, not just his individual parts. Therefore, primarily homœopathy has less appeal for the man of mechanical bent, for it is this man who makes the best surgeon. Instead, homœopathy offers a gentler way toward health of the entire individual.

One thing the student must consider is the differentiation between medicine and public health service. Public health service, ideally, has to do with the prevention of disease in the community, in guarding food and water supplies, in providing facilities and restrictions for adequate healthy housing conditions and in attending to the proper disposal of waste matter, so that the health of the community will be guarded against epidemics borne by impure water, milk or other food supplies, or born in insanitary or unhygienic conditions.

Medicine ideally has to do with the cure of disease, the building up of the individual, not overlooking the proper hygiene and sanitation, but with a deeper view of the needs of the individual himself, rather than the needs of the community.

Homœopathic medicine goes even further than this, for homœopathy seeks to relieve the individual as much as possible from the heavy burden of the hereditary tendencies he carries, and to guard against increasing this load by enabling his vital energy to provide its own immunity against disease. Homœopathy looks upon the health of the individual as a precious charge, and the return of the individual to health as almost certain if we but follow the fundamental laws.

Another growing distinction between public health service, so called, and medicine, especially homœopathic medicine, is the increasing use of serums and vaccines. It has been claimed that these preparations are really homœopathic ; even instructors in the homœopathic colleges have thought thus to demonstrate homœopathic principles. Let the young man consider this logically.

In the first place, giving the *identical* instead of the *similar* means the difference between isopathy and homœopathy. You may say that the *identical*, in the case of the serum or vaccine, is potentiated, somewhat as in homœopathy, and therefore removes it from the identical sphere. Although potentiated, it does not alter the fact that it was not in the first place similar, but identical. In the second place, it has been potentiated in mass production, and potentiated and filtered, not through an inert substance, but through living creatures, and a lower order of creatures at that.

There is a biological law that crossing the blood of a higher and lower order of creatures means destruction to the species, and it is well to consider this. Practically, we may well look to the nature of growth in different orders of creatures. When an animal has a longevity of some twenty years and in that time attains a weight of half a ton, there must be a rapid cell growth. When serum from such a source, though ever so highly filtered, is injected into the human race, where normal longevity is seventy years and where 160 pounds might be considered an average weight, one can well understand the impact upon the vital energy of the human ; for while the serum is considered by ordinary medicine to be potentiated past all danger, homœopathy believes that potentiation in any or all forms means a more prompt release of power than may have been possible in the normal state, it then being latent.

One of the outstanding problems to-day is cancer. It intrigues the mind of the young man, and his search for the cause and cure of cancer is indefatigable. This is a challenge to the homœopathic physician as well, since he has remedial aids that ordinary practice knows not ; but let the young man consider this problem in the light of public health service and its insistence on the use of serums and vaccines. Let him weigh his ability to stand upon his adherence to fundamental principles. If he takes up the task on the frontier of cancer study, will he remember the relationship between homœopathy (not isopathy) and disease conditions, or will he forget that human cell tissue is easily stimulated to overgrowth, under certain hereditary tendencies ? He has here a field for work which offers much elbow room and all the dangers of the pioneer.

The homœopathic school accentuates the study of the action of drugs upon healthy human beings, with little consideration of their action on the lower animals, for homœopathy recognizes that it is only through a knowledge of their action on man that we can obtain a correct perception of their applicability in disease. The field here is ripe for much investigation, and the results of such investigation would enrich the homœopathic materia medica by completing provings of some of the older remedies, and by bringing out provings of new remedies. This is an opportunity that only homœopathy offers, for the teaching of remedy reaction has ceased in ordinary medical colleges.

The decision lies with the individual, and what he is determined to secure from his life work. If it is financial

2

ambition, he had better not take up homœopathy. Homœopathy is a principle, and principles brook no division of
loyalty. If he has at heart the desire to serve, he may find
fame and riches at his door as well as that keen satisfaction
of knowing that he has brought to his clientele the gift of
healing in the safest, gentlest and most rapid manner.

For the man who can help the community, as individuals,
toward a higher level of health, the community has a place
of honour ; for the man who can assist Nature to cure
serious illness a certain fame in the community there is
burning, perhaps not the bright flame of the comet, but a
steady glow of light for his path. For the man who spends
himself unceasingly for those about him the community will
return a comfortable livelihood, not the spectacular fortune
offered in some lines of endeavour, but a competence which
will enable him to keep his family in a well-earned place in
the community.

Homœopathy as a profession carries a challenge. The
possibilities of its art are infinite.

What future has homœopathy to offer to you ? Young
man, what have you to offer homœopathy ?

CHAPTER II

INTRODUCTION TO THE STUDY OF HOMŒOPATHY

IF a physician would successfully practise medicine he must know, first, what is curable by medicine, and second, what is curative in drugs.

The physician must know something of the history of the development of the drug action ; of the gradual experiments with the remedial substance upon healthy human beings and the data gathered therefrom over a long period of careful observations, which have been checked and verified again and again, both in experimental provings and in clinical use. The basis upon which this knowledge of drug action is built is a profound and basic element of homœopathic procedure.

By the time the physician has become somewhat acquainted with these guides he is in a position to go forward and erect the structure of his future medical career upon a basis that is immovable, that does not change with every new theory that arises upon the medical horizon. If we look thoughtfully at medical literature over a period of years we find it one kaleidoscopic panorama of ever-changing theory and practice.

Homœopathy, on the other hand, is ever capable of development, while the principles remain the same. Homœopathy is founded upon principles that are again founded upon natural laws. These natural laws are basic, they are more eternal than the hills, for these laws were formulated before the hills came into being.

If a man follows where homœopathy leads he must be able to follow those laws and to hold close to them, regardless of pressure or influence. On the other hand, the very principles which he follows stabilize him and make him sure in his work. This stability can be maintained equally well in chronic work, in acute cases or amidst the panics of epidemics of unknown origin, such as influenza, poliomyelitis ; outbreaks of such conditions as encephalitis ; for here, as in all other manifestations of illness, the fundamental laws remain firm and intact, and they are sufficiently basic to provide a sure guide to health. A man who adopts the homœopathic methods must be free from prejudice, and able to look fairly at disease conditions from a new angle. He must look at the patient as an individual, not as a disease, and he must treat the patient, not the disease. He must learn that the symptoms that under ordinary training would have been discarded as confusing the issue or as of no value are the very symptoms which, to the homœopathic physician, simplify the case and provide the strongest clues to the surest method of assistance.

He must possess a sense of values, and be able to train himself to observe and interpret those signs which manifest themselves through the habits and circumstances of the patient, into indications for health-restoring medication which he has at his command.

In other words, he must learn to observe and record cases from the homœopathic angle. The diagnostic viewpoint which has featured so largely in his training must here take a different place in his perspective. He must take time to trace the source of the disturbance and the remedy to fit the complete picture, always basing the process upon the sound rock of natural laws.

Homœopathy opens up a vista of opportunities for continually seeking new fields for the demonstration of natural laws, for if, as we believe, these laws are fundamental, their application is universal, and had we the vision to see it we would be convinced not from its application in the field of medicine alone, but in every field of natural science and in applied science as well.

The vista in the field of medicine which is opened up for cure under the homœopathic method of treatment is a wide one, and cure is always accomplished with the least possible disturbance to the patient and in the gentlest manner, yet with the most profound effect on the whole individual. Homœopathy is a system of medicine upon which we can depend to set the individual system in order, and the patient on the high road to recovery, if recovery is possible. If we fail, we may know that the failure is ours, in that we have not fully compassed the case or a knowledge of the remedies. In a field so vast, it is conceivable that not all available agencies have yet been developed ; and our own ignorance may limit us in the use of those remedies which we already have, but those who study homœopathy with an unprejudiced mind, and those who have practised it faithfully and purely, can and do attest its unsurpassed results when conscientiously applied to the sick.

If a chain is no stronger than its weakest link, we must examine the links individually, one by one, and not determine their strength or weakness by testing the complete chain as our first measure.

The very foundation of homœopathic practice considers man not only as an individual, but as a complete unit in himself, of which all his parts comprise a well-balanced whole. Homœopathy, therefore, does not consider any one part as being ill, but considers the manifestation of illness in one part in its relation to the whole man.

Medicine ideally has to do with the cure of disease, the building up of the individual, not overlooking proper hygiene and sanitation, but with a deeper view of the needs of the individual himself, once again considering his individuality. Probably homœopathy stresses this view of the individual in relation to his environment and circumstances more than any other school of medical thought, for it takes into consideration not only his immediate heritage, but the more subtle and complex burden that is the heritage of long ages of struggling and developing ancestors. Homœopathy seeks to relieve the individual as much as possible from the heavy burden of hereditary tendencies he carries, and to guard against increasing this load by enabling his vital energy to provide its own immunity against disease. Homœopathy looks upon the health of the individual as a precious charge, and his return to health as almost certain if we but follow the fundamental laws.

Homœopathy accentuates the study of the action of drugs upon healthy human beings, with little consideration of their action on the lower animals, for homœopathy recognizes that it is only through a knowledge of their action upon man that we can obtain a correct perception of their applicability in disease. This is a field in which homœopathy leads all other forms of medical thought, for no school of medicine has carried on, over such a long period of years, such intensive study of remedy reaction, nor has any such extensive experimental work been done with the results so faithfully recorded by such a large group of people, with the results so carefully checked by clinical application.

This can truly be designated as scientific, for the results have been checked and rechecked, and the findings applied with unfailing success when the proper principles were followed.

The generally accepted concept of homœopathy is that it is concerned chiefly with the law of similars. Indeed, the encyclopædia gives as the definition of homœopathy that it is a system of medicine based upon the law of similars. While for a concentrated definition this might serve, yet there is much more to homœopathy than the law of similars, for it would be very incomplete did it not embrace much more than this. It might better be defined as a system of medicine based upon natural laws.

We need to get a more complete and comprehensive insight into the scope of these laws. There is danger of making a fetish of the faith in homœopathy by expecting wonderful results where a proper understanding of these laws would deter us from attempting the use of homœopathy. Sometimes even without a knowledge of these laws we obtain wonderful results, it is true, but we often fail by not carrying out the teaching of Hahnemann, to remove the cause of the disease where it is manifestly a mechanical trouble. Again, in the class of diseases where malnutrition results from lack of the proper foods, instead of the lack of powers of assimilation, homœopathy cannot be expected to take the place of the proper elements in the diet.

On the other hand, in the field of therapeutics by curative medicine there is no other absolutely curative assistance. Here homœopathic laws reign supreme. To confuse the scope of each of these fields makes for misunderstanding and failure.

Homœopathy considers the morbid vital processes in

living organisms, which are perceptibly represented by symptoms, irrespective of what caused them. Homœopathy is concerned only with disease *per se*, that is, in its primary, functional, or dynamic aspect, not in its ultimate and so-called pathological results. With these we have nothing to do ; these are not in any sense the disease but are the results of disease conditions. Therefore we must distinguish between the primary functional symptoms which represent the morbid process itself, and the secondary symptoms which represent the pathological end products of disease.

The gross physical pathology such as we find in gallstones we do not prescribe for, but we do prescribe for the patient, being guided by the symptoms which began in the perversion of the vital process, which preceded and accompanied the ultimate development of the gallstones.

Functional symptoms always precede structural changes. In biology, " function creates and develops the organ ". In disease, function, the effort of the vital energy to function under adverse circumstances, precedes and develops the pathological states. For the homœopathic physician the totality of the functional symptoms of the patient is the disease and constitutes the only perceptible form of disease, and therefore the only basis of curative treatment. Symptoms are the outward and visible signs of the inward disturbance of the vital force which will ultimately produce morbid states, and when these symptoms are removed the disease ceases to exist.

Homœopathy is not concerned with the morbific agents any more than it is with the tangible products or the ultimates of disease. Hahnemann regarded the removal of all obstacles to cure as absolutely essential before he attempted to proceed to the selection and administration of the remedy which was homœopathic to the symptoms of the individual case, by which alone the cure is to be accomplished.

We thus focus our attention upon the individual and purely functional side of disease, upon disease itself, where we can perceive the sphere of homœopathy. Thus from this view disease is a constant change of functions and transformations so long as life lasts. We are here dealing in the realm of pure dynamics. This field is the field of disordered vital energy, and therefore disordered vital ·expressions and functional changes in the individual patient, irrespective of the name of the disease or its cause, and is governed by the laws of motion in the vital realm. It is in this sphere that vital functions act—in the realm of the laws of Mutual Action : ACTION AND REACTION ARE EQUAL AND OPPOSITE.

In his *Organon*, Par. 6, Hahnemann says :

The unprejudiced observer, well aware of the futility of transcendental speculation which can receive no confirmation from experience—be his power of penetration never so great—takes note of nothing in every individual disease, except the *changes* in the health of the body and the mind (morbid phenomena, accidents, symptoms) which can be perceived externally by means of the senses ; that is to say, he notices only the deviations from a former healthy state of the diseased individual, which are felt by the patient himself, remarked by those around him and observed by the physician. All these perceptible signs represent the disease in its whole extent, that is, together they form the true and only conceivable portrait of the disease.

Disease itself is impossible of observation ; we only see and record the effects of disease ; we can only record the symptoms. Disease is as elusive as thought ; we are utterly unable to discern thoughts, save such as are transformed into acts ; so we only recognize disease as it is made manifest in symptoms. The inner expressions are dynamic in nature, their outward expression is functional. While all this is true, yet we are dealing with the most positive of facts—for symptoms are a record of facts—facts registered in symptoms are the most exact record of the expression of the vital energy to the morbific agent.

Once more to quote Hahnemann's *Organon* :

There must be a curative principle present in medicine ; reason divines as much. But its inner nature is in no way to be perceived by us ; its mode of expression and its outward effects alone can be judged by experience.

Health is restored after the removal of all symptoms ; then and only then is all disease removed. Hahnemann this way distinguishes between disease itself and its causes, manifestations, and products, and then shows at once that the sphere of homœopathy is limited to functional changes from which the phenomena of diseases arise. Thus homœopathy operates only in the dynamic sphere. Directly, homœopathy has nothing in common with the physical cause or product of disease, but secondarily it is related. Here is the place where surgery may have its function, yet many of the tangible effects may remain. If these effects are too far advanced, they may be removed. If this is not done, it stands to reason that the best effects of the remedy will not be realized, but we must differentiate between the causes of disease and the ultimates of disease ; they stand at opposite ends of the scale. While these ultimates are not primarily within the range of *similia*, and therefore not the objective of homœopathic treatment, the morbid process from which they arise or to which they lead is under the control of homœopathic medication. This medication may control and retard the development of pathological conditions. Thus tumours may be retarded or completely arrested, and absorption increased, and finally the disappearance of the growth ; secretions or excretions increased or decreased ; ulcers healed ; but all this is secondary to the real cure which takes place solely in the dynamic sphere, restoring the patient to health and harmonious functioning of his whole being by the dynamic influence of the symptomatically similar remedy.

As Stuart Close has well said, the real field of homœopathy is

To those agents which effect the organism as to health in ways not governed by chemistry, mechanics, or hygiene, but those capable of producing ailments similar to those found in the sick.

Fincke has shown that in the development and growth of the child much can be done to make this symmetrical, for it is closely related to the laws of assimilation ; here the laws of *similia* have pre-eminence, for the child is peculiarly under the influence of the laws of action and reaction as applied to the action of the similar remedy in its development and growth.

The homœopathic principle is not used in another field of

what might be called extreme emergency, but rather we use what may be called a principle of palliation. As Hahnemann says in a note to Par. 67 of the *Organon* :

Only in the most urgent cases, where danger to life and imminent death allow no time for the action of a homœopathic remedy—not hours, sometimes not even quarter hours and scarcely minutes—in sudden accidents occurring to previously healthy individuals—for example, in asphyxia and suspended animation from lightning, from suffocation, freezing, drowning, etc.—it is admissible and even judicious at all events as a preliminary measure to stimulate the irritability and sensibility (the physical life) with a palliative, as for instance, gentle electric shocks, with clysters of strong coffee, with a stimulating odour, gradual applications of heat, etc. When this stimulation is effected, the play of vital organs goes on again in its former healthy manner, for here there is no disease to be removed, but merely an obstruction and suppression to the healthy vital force. To this category belong various antidotes to sudden poisonings : alkalis for mineral acids, hepar sulphuris for metallic poisons, coffee and camphor (and ipecacuanha) for poisoning by opium, etc.

Even in emergencies, however, we may find the indications for the homœopathic remedy just as clear-cut as antipathic means would be, and if we can read these indications, even here the action of the potentized remedy will be more rapid and far more gentle in its restorative powers than would be the case if stronger measures were taken. Thus in such conditions as asphyxia, shock from various sources, and even from the ingestion of poisons, among many other so-called emergencies, homœopathic remedies in skilful hands have saved lives with almost miraculous speed and with the happiest of results. The indicated remedy works with exceeding rapidity, and we dare not put a limitation upon its restorative powers.

It is well to obtain this clear view of what is before us and face candidly the true place for the practice of the healing art that we may become true physicians ; and to stabilize still further, let us look at what Carroll Dunham called *the scientific reasonableness of homœopathy.*

Homœopathy has been developed through the inductive method of reasoning. Not only are the conclusions cᶠ homœopathy consistent with its assumption but they are founded upon Truth, for homœopathy as a method is drawn logically according to the strictest rules of inductive generalization from data derived from the closest observation of facts and experiments. All the processes from the proving to the curative prescription are controlled by the principles of inductive reasoning.

Funk & Wagnall's *Dictionary* defines inductive reasoning as follows :

The Inductive Method in Reasoning is the scientific method that proceeds by induction. It requires (1) *exact observation* : (2) *correct interpretation* of the observed facts with a view to understanding them in relation to each other and their causes ; (3) *rational explanation* of the facts by referring them to their real cause or law ; and (4) *scientific construction* : putting the facts in such co-ordination that the system reached shall agree with the reality.

Let us examine the earliest steps taken by Hahnemann in his development of the scientific approach toward the healing of the sick through the reasonable application of natural laws.

His childhood training in logical thinking crystallized his keen mind and made him peculiarly fitted for the task he assumed. In other words, he was early trained in inductive reasoning, and he was able to scientifically construct hitherto unknown principles in the care of the sick.

(1) *Exact observation* : Hahnemann's honest disappointment with the practice of medicine as manifested in the eighteenth century was the direct result of his faculties of observation and reasoning. His early training demanded of him that he find logical reasons for the administration of medicinal substances, and that once given, favourable results were to be expected.

The chaotic prescriptions of that day left little reasonable grounds for clear-cut results, and his observations of the frequent failure of the physician to help sick patients toward cure, or worse still, the rapid decline of the patient in seemingly simple and uncomplicated cases under the best medical care procurable, led Hahnemann to renounce the practice of medicine. He turned to chemistry and the translation of medical literature as a means of livelihood. In one of these translations an item on the use of cinchona bark for intermittent fever arrested his attention, since he himself had recently suffered such a malady. His interest was aroused, and his experiments with medicinal substances (which he later called *provings*) were begun.

Here he first caught the gleam of light that led him to an understanding of the reasonable application of remedies, based on the *exact observation* of the ability of the drug to produce symptoms, on the one hand, and of the symptoms of the patient on the other. This problem he simplified to a logical basis.

(2) *Correct interpretation* of the phenomena produced by the experiments or provings was provided by close study of series of these experiments on groups of people. Thus the probability of error was reduced through the accumulation of more data, with increasingly exact observation not only of results produced, but of possible interposing conditions which varied the results.

Hahnemann was soon convinced that (3) the *rational explanation* of the phenomena was the thought, hinted at in the time of the ancient Hindu sages, by Hippocrates, Paracelsus, Stahl and others throughout the course of medical history, that " diseases are cured by medicines that have the power to excite a similar affection ".

While this thought had been applied occasionally, Hahnemann was the first to insist on the importance of this premise in every case where a true cure was achieved, as he was the first to test remedial substances and classify the results with this purpose in mind.

With (4) true *scientific construction* he applied the principles evolved from his inductive reasoning and the correlating experiments he had conducted.

Briefly, then, we find that these experiments had led Hahnemann to give a medicinal substance to healthy persons, to carefully record the effects—which were the production of symptoms of (artificial) disease—for the purpose of making these substances available for people suffering from like symptoms in (natural) disease syndromes. Thus developed his thorough work in proving as we know it.

This hypothesis, a process of inductive reasoning, proved to be a triumph through the discovery of scientific principles based on natural laws.

So, too, the principles of inductive reasoning led Hahnemann, through his observation of the effects of remedies administered on the basis of symptom similarity, to the gradual decrease of the dose, because of the consequent drug effects (as differentiated from the remedial effects) of the substances administered. This decrease of the dose was developed according to a definitely scaled formula, and this in turn led to a discovery of the principle of potentiation, or release of energy.

This discovery of the principle of potentization was Hahnemann's greatest gift to science in general, and to medicine in particular. Had it not been for his powers of observation and his interpretation of those observations through rational explanation, and his action upon those observations, he would never have achieved this eminence. When we consider the centuries of medical practice that preceded Hahnemann, and the years of medical practice and scientific research that have followed, and comprehend somewhat the significance of his discovery of powers released through minute division, we can but marvel at his keen logic and strive to follow his processes of reasoning.

Thus we readily see and appreciate the aptitude of Stuart Close's description of homœopathy, when he describes the foundations as " solid concrete, composed of the broken rock of hard facts, united by the cement of a great natural principle . . . " upon which the superstructure has been raised so soundly that it is inseparable from the foundation.

This shows the relation of facts to the practice of homœopathy, with an outline of the reasoning process by which homœopathy was worked out and built up ; and it is applicable in every concrete case which a homœopathic physician may be called upon to treat. The principles involved are the same : the examination of the patient, or the record of the proving ; the analysis and evaluation of the symptoms in each case ; the selection of the remedy ; all these are conducted under the rules and in an orderly·

method based upon inductive reasoning. Thus we determine what is characteristic in the patient and in the remedy ; the characteristic symptoms are always the generals of the patient.

What is true of one symptom may often be true of the whole patient, as illustrated by the reaction to thermic changes of individual parts and symptoms, and may be true of the whole man ; therefore, while we strive to form a picture of the totality of the symptoms, we must instinctively evaluate, and find ourselves assembling symptoms as applying to the whole man or to his individual parts, as the case may be. As Close well puts it, in his *Genius of Homœopathy* :

Logic facilitates the comprehension of the related totality or picture of the symptoms of the case as a whole. From all the parts, logic constructs the whole. It reveals the case ; in other words, by generalizing it assigns each detail to its proper place and gives concrete form to the case so that it may be grasped by the mind in its entirety.

The true " totality " is more than the mere numerical totality or whole number of the symptoms. It may even exclude some of the particular symptoms if they cannot, at the time, be logically related to the case. Such symptoms are called " accidental symptoms ", and are not allowed to influence the choice of the remedy. The " totality " is that concrete form which the symptoms take when they are logically related to each other and stand forth as an individuality, recognizable by anyone who is familiar with the symptomatic forms and lineaments of drugs and diseases.

The basis of the homœopathic prescription is the totality of the symptoms of the patient, *as viewed and interpreted from the standpoint of the prescriber.* A successful prescription cannot be made from the standpoint of the diagnostician, the surgeon nor the pathologist, as such, because of the differing interpretation and classification of symptoms. *A prescription can only be made upon those symptoms which have their counterpart or similar in the materia medica.*

Individuality is inculcated always in the examination of a case. The three steps always followed in a carefully developed case consist in the examination of the patient, the examination of the symptom record of the patient, and the examination of the materia medica.

After these steps are logically taken and analysed they lead by the process of induction to the generals of the case, for the generals are the sum total of the particulars. The value of the generalization depends primarily upon the data from which it is drawn, for it is an axiom of philosophy that " a general truth is but the aggregate of particular truths, a comprehensive expression by which an indefinite number of individual facts are affirmed or denied ".

It is not possible to form generals until we have considered special particular symptoms and analysed and assimilated them, in their relation to the whole. Minor particulars enter into major, and majors into one all-inclusive concept of the case. Such an all-inclusive major is *similia similibus curantur*—the most complete and far-reaching generalization ever made from the deduction of individual facts.

The value of generalization depends in its essence upon the data from which it is drawn. The facts must be both accurate and complete.

Where we have many and clear mental symptoms they are always generals, for they represent the man in the most characteristic sense. Modalities again are always generals, for they are the natural modifiers of the case. " Where there are no generals," says Kent, " we can expect no cures."

The approach to the study of the case and the approach to the study of the materia medica are essentially the same— the materia medica is the *facsimile* of the sickness.

Bœnninghausen has shown in his repertory that these aggravations and ameliorations are modalities and therefore rank as generals. Close rates this repertorial work as " the greatest masterpiece of analysis, comparison and generalization in our literature " The attempt to limit the application of the modality to the particular symptoms with which they were first observed has not been successful in practice, so Bœnninghausen's grouping of them as generals was a masterpiece of inductive reasoning. Writing in regard to these modalities which he considers generals, he says :

All of these indications are so trustworthy, and have been verified by such manifold experiences that hardly any others can equal them in rank; to say nothing of surpassing them. But the most valuable fact respecting them is this : That this characteristic is not confined to one or another symptom, *but like a red thread it runs through all the morbid symptoms of a given remedy, which are associated with any kind of pain whatever,* or even with a sensation of discomfort, and hence it is available for both external and internal symptoms of the most varied character.

He arrived at these truths by the inductive study of the facts, and the results were the products of sound reasoning.

We see, then, that homœopathy is more than the law of similars. It is basically a scientific method of healing which is based upon natural laws and developed by inductive reasoning. It is closely allied with the principles of natural growth and development. The whole fabric is summed up in the third paragraph of the *Organon,* where Hahnemann writes :

If the physician clearly perceives what it is' in disease in general and in each case of disease in particular that has to be cured (knowledge of disease, knowledge of the requirements of disease or disease-indications) : if he clearly perceives what is the healing principle in medicine generally and in each medicine in particular (knowledge of the powers of medicines) : if in the light of clear principles he can so adapt the healing virtue of the drug to the illness that is to be cured that recovery must follow, and if he has the ability not only to select the particular remedy whose mode of action is most suitable for the case (choice of the remedy or indicated medicine), but also to choose the exact quantity of the remedy required (the suitable dose) and the fitting period for its repetition, if, I say, he knows all these things and in addition recognizes in every case the hindrances to lasting recovery and can remove them, *then truly he understands how to build up his work on an adequate basis of reason, and he is a rational practitioner of the healing art.*

What must a physician know before he can successfully practise medicine ? (*Answer :* What is curable by medicine and what is curative in drugs.)

How can he learn what is curative in drugs ?

Compare the value of homœopathy in chronic and acute work.

How does the homœopathic physician regard seemingly confusing symptoms ?

In what relationship does homœopathy consider the sickness of local parts ?

Why does homœopathy not give more weight to the experimentation upon the lower animals ?

Why do we feel that the knowledge of drugs and their reaction, assembled and recorded by homœopathy, is truly scientific ?

What is the larger definition of homœopathy ? (*Answer :* A system of medicine based upon natural laws.)

How does homœopathy regard gross physical pathology ?

What did Hahnemann mean by " removing all obstacles to cure " ?

How does disease manifest itself ?

How much can we ever learn of disease ?

How do we treat emergencies, such as poisoning, asphyxia, etc ?

What do we mean by natural disease ?   By artificial disease ?

CHAPTER III

VITAL FORCE

THERE is much misapprehension about homœopathy among physicians as well as among the laity. Among physicians there is a feeling that if we know the materia medica that is all that is required. The materia medica is indeed important, and its thorough comprehension and study is needed at all times ; but unless the homœopathic physician has a concept of the philosophy, of the reasons underlying the administration of the remedy, he will never make a careful homœopathic physician.

The study of the materia medica by Hahnemann would have caused no disturbance among the medical men of his day ; it was when Hahnemann taught his fundamental principles that he drew forth antagonism and ire as against a new and revolutionary (and therefore dangerous) doctrine. So in order to understand homœopathy, and to get the proper concept of administering our remedies, and even of taking the case and eliciting symptoms, we must get Hahnemann's concept of the principles that enter into the studies of the homœopathic physician.

One of the first and foremost elements with which the homœopathic physician must be conversant is the different forms of energy, for it is on this basis only that we can prescribe homœopathically. In Hahnemann's *Organon of the Healing Art* he gives us the following :

In the healthy condition of man the spirit-like vital force, the dynamis that animates the material body, rules with unbounded sway and retains all the parts of the organism in admirable harmonious vital operation as regards both sensations and functions, so that our indwelling, reason-gifted mind can freely employ this living, healthy instrument for the higher purposes of our existence.

This was the first introduction to the medical world of the rational concept of life itself.

We recognize life in three parts, the body, the mind, and the spirit. This is a trinity, and this trinity is always present in all life and in some form in every part of our organism. These forces react in sympathy and are interdependent. (Vide *Organon* 43.)

No organ, no tissue, no cell, no molecule, is independent of the activities of the others, but the life of each one of these elements is merged into the life of the whole. The unit of human life cannot be the organ, the tissue, the cell, the molecule, the atom, but the whole organism, the whole man.

We are prone to think of attained life as composed of these three members which make it a trinity, but we must remember also that life is a unity from its inception. When the two parent cells are united that vital principle, the vital energy, is already present ; and the ego of the completed cell does not change one iota after once beginning its process; it has in itself and of itself the power to develop the cells, the physical, because of the continual flowing through them of the vital energy which dominates the whole. It has within itself the power to develop muscle, nerve, brain—cells individual in themselves, gifted with the powers for specialized uses in the future. Yet these are all a part of the whole man ; and while we have in each individual infinite powers of development, unless the ego in its initial stage is energized and capable of development, it will never grow to its highest capacity. Without this vital energy, the cell, or the whole body, becomes inanimate and is dead. It is only when the vital energy is present that there is a living organism, capable of physical action and of the exercise of mental powers and the ability to take hold on the spiritual forces.

No two individuals are alike. The development of the vital energy in one differs from that in another. Each one possesses a special personality and a special psychophysical construction which is determined by the interplay of hereditary tendencies and factors of disease.

The growth and development of each individual progresses as it draws upon the physical energy, and upon the dynamic energy as it is manifest in the brain, and upon the spiritual energy. These different manifestations of energy are essentially different in their workings. The law of growth is the same in one as in another. The mingling of these expressions of energy is the united personality, and when the energy functions properly in all the three manifestations the whole personality grows harmoniously, for the energy is the power house that supplies the impetus of growth for the whole economy, the whole individual. When the energy functions improperly there is greater growth on one plane than on another and the personality is not symmetrical in its development.

The nature of energy is dynamic, and this dynamis penetrates every particle, every cell, every atom of the human economy. Any disturbance of this vital energy or force results in a disfigured or disturbed development of the whole human economy. Such a disturbance may come from pre-natal influences, such as the effects of sudden fright ; it may be caused by indulgences on the part of either or both parents at the time of conception ; the cause may lie in excessive worry during gestation ; it may be due to hereditary stigma of either one or both of the parent cells, which may perhaps be due to hereditary diseases or miasms. Like an indelible brand, the warping of this dynamic energy is a stain that " will not out ".

On the other hand, after the separate individual life has been established, we know how terrific are the consequences of fright : the fright of the mother who transmits the effects to the nursing child, with a consequent disturbance to the vital energy long after the incident is forgotten. Or the mother's vital force may be disturbed by worries, or by sudden fright, and she herself may suffer from the consequent serious disturbance. These are but a few instances where there may be serious disturbances of the vital force.

The influence of this vital force on the whole organism is so delicately adjusted and so intimately connected with every part, that seemingly distant organs or unrelated symptoms show the effects of any disturbance of the vital force ; and no one can prophesy what the influence may be on the part of the economy or what direction will be taken by the manifestations in each individual, but his vital energy will direct the course with unerring precision.

The appearance of these disturbances is a reflection of the inward turmoil and confusion of the harmonious action which the vital force has suffered. This brings us to the point where we must acknowledge that disturbance of any part is the manifestation of an inner disturbance and is not a local confusion of certain muscles or of certain groups of nerves, or arteries, or even of the mind itself ; but that it is an expression of the whole disturbance manifesting itself perhaps locally or in seemingly unrelated parts ; it is an expression of the disturbed vital energy, and is a manifestation of the man as a unit, and not of the separate parts of his body. That brings us to the point of looking upon disease as a dynamic expression of the disturbance of the harmony and rhythm of the vital energy. That rhythm may be so disturbed as to increase the pace or to lower the vitality, and that in itself either raises or lowers the reactions of the body and of the mind and of the spirit. They are all united under the supreme mastery of the vital energy.

In treating disease we are drawing also upon another storehouse of dynamic force, which acts almost synchronously with the disturbed vital force that is in the body. The pace is similar, the symptoms are similar. We are dealing with the similar remedy. Dr. Boger illustrates this by the picture of the runaway train, where an engine is sent, not in the opposite direction to meet and combat force with force, but in the same direction, increasing in pace until it is equal in pace to the runaway ; and it is then in a position to subdue its speed.

Disease symptoms show themselves in unified order in the physical, the mental and the spiritual spheres, but each individual does not show necessarily disturbances in all of these spheres in manifesting diseased conditions. One, the insane, may accentuate the mental ; one the physical ; and one, the criminal, the disturbance of the spiritual forces ; each is accentuated according to the tendencies of the vital energy and the individual reaction to the dynamic disturbance.

Any disturbance of this vital energy immediately shows itself in lack of harmony through the outward manifestations of our beings ; in other words, symptoms. When harmonious functioning is disturbed, we get sickness as a result, and it has as its base and inception this lack of harmony in the flow of vital energy through the body. This is manifest in disease as it naturally develops because of disturbed vital force, and it develops also in disturbed vital force from the proving of remedies, showing the action of remedies and the very nature of the remedies themselves.

This is the reason why the remedies are potentized so that they may reach more surely the vital energy of the individual. Were they not in potential form they would not reach the vital energy as promptly and directly, and it is a question whether they would not be in a toxic form which would destroy or subvert the vital energy without showing the proper symptomatology. The best provings that we have, showing the finer differentiations and the most pronounced reaction, are made from the potencies from the 30th upward, because it is in this form that they more readily meet the vital energy as it pervades the whole organism, and they create reactions that are not capable of being produced in the cruder exhibitions, which are largely toxic.

The action of the proven remedy is similar to the action of disease from whatever source. Disease first must be caused by a disturbance of the vital energy and that in itself sets in motion a train of symptoms exhibiting an exact picture of the way in which the vital energy is disturbed. It is only from these pictures that we can gather an understanding of the inner workings of the sick individual. It is only through the careful observation of the provings of the potencies that we can know the action of any given remedy, to understand where it has made its impress on the vital force. The vital force is resilient and impressions not only show forth promptly but over a considerable period of time, and in orderly groups of symptoms, even as does natural disease.

Organon, Pars. 10, 11 :

The material organism, without the vital force, is capable of no sensation, no function, no self-preservation ; it derives all sensation and performs all the functions of life solely by means of the immaterial being (the vital force) which animates the material organism in health and in disease.

When a person falls ill it is only this spiritual, self-acting (automatic) vital force, everywhere present in the organism, that is primarily deranged by the dynamic influence upon it of a morbific agent inimical to life ; it is only the vital force, deranged to such an abnormal state, that can furnish the organism with its disagreeable sensations and incline it to the irregular processes which we call disease ; for, as a power invisible in itself, and only cognizable by its effects on the organism, its morbid derangement only makes itself known by the manifestation of disease in the sensations and functions of those parts of the organism exposed to the senses of the observer and physician ; that is, by morbid symptoms, and in no other way can it make itself known.

This brings us to a consideration of the unhampered expression of the vital force and its influence in disease and cure. As we have seen, its expression reflects the exact symptoms of the disturbance. One of the easiest methods of dealing with sickness is to give medicines or mechanical treatments which put a stop to the symptoms ; however, this is more apt to further upset the vital force by suppressing the individual expression of the disordered vital energy. Anything that disturbs the normal expression of disturbed harmony simply adds to the disturbance that is already in existence, and is a confusion worse confounded, for it suppresses or distorts the manifestations of the diseased state. This may be done in many ways. It may be done by sprays ; it may be done by ointments ; it may be done by irritative or narcotic treatment. Whatever is done that interferes with the expression of the disturbance as is manifested by the symptomatology of the patient adds many fold to our troubles. The altered character or entire suppression of discharges ; the suppression of eruptions ; the palliation of pain by narcotics ; the momentary invigoration by tonics ; these are among our problems. The injections in gonorrhœa, for instance, may suppress the discharge, but the effect is to throw the whole vital energy out of balance more markedly than before, and we get all kinds of manifestations in distant and seemingly unrelated organs as a result. Suppression is the easiest and greatest of the errors that can be practised by any graduate in medicine.

To what did Hahnemann attribute the harmonious functioning of the human organism ?

What is the unit of human life ?

What do we mean by the trinity of the individual ?

Cite some conditions that may cause disturbance of the vital force with consequent disturbed development of the whole economy.

What is the outward reflection of the inward turmoil ?

Why do we look on disease as a dynamic expression rather than as a local matter ?

Why do we speak of the dynamic force of remedies ?

What is sickness ?   (*Answer :* Disturbance of harmonious functions.)

Why are remedies potentized ?

What is the effect of suppressive treatment in disease conditions ?

CHAPTER IV

VITAL FORCE AS EXPRESSED IN FUNCTIONS: IN HEALTH, IN DISEASE, IN RECOVERY, IN CURE

THE life and composition of cells is of a complex nature. The composition of animal protoplasm is capable of analysis, yet there is in each cell and its life function that which is beyond our comprehension and defies analysis. We cannot as yet fathom the reason why a human ovum takes on growth and development only when the spermatozoa imbeds itself deep in its innermost nuclei. We only know that it possesses some hidden vital function that compels it to develop and grow. The power of each life to develop from the single ovum into its own ego, unfolding and expressing itself for ever in its own way and individuality, never varying from the ideal that is once stamped, to carry out to its perfection all the powers of adult life, distinguishing it from all other created species, is a marvel until we comprehend the principle of the vital force or energy permeating all created things. That power, although defying analysis, nevertheless continues all through life as a mysterious manifestation of the vital functions. It is the close study of these vital functions that becomes the chief study of the physician.

In order to obtain a thorough knowledge of these vital functions we must study them in their manifestations during health. From the earliest period of its existence growth is manifest from within the cell out; it is never observed growing from without in. The one point most vital to observe is the course and direction of its expression—always from within outward. This is true in the embryonic state and is always maintained as long as life exists. This is equally true in the specialization of functions. The special organs are developed and their functions maintained by the expression of the vital energy as the life-giving principle. All expressions of the mind are such manifestations. Indeed, it is the expression of the vital force in and through the mind and intellect that has a very great influence in the functioning of all life and of the special organs.

In health all expressions of vital force may be expressed by perfect functioning of all parts of the body and by a sense of general well-being.

In disease this expression is vastly changed. There is a sense of discomfort. The mental expressions are vastly altered according to the degree of disturbance. Physical signs and symptoms appear ; and all because the vital functions are disturbed either from external impressions having a depressing effect, and the consequent reaction of the vital force, or from some hidden miasm coming into its full expression in its impress on the vital force. External impressions having a profound effect upon the vital force are such circumstances as the shock of sudden news, either bad news or joyful news ; or severe fright, such as the "shell-shock " we see with our soldiers ; long mental and physical strains ; and various other reactions. All of these external forces, when in conjunction with an already disturbed vital force, have very profound effects upon the vital functions and they are manifested in a trail of symptoms which are expressed in different ways in varying individuals.

Likewise the vital function in its manifestations often shows the effect of inherited miasms and dyscrasias, where the protozoon has become vitiated by disease processes in the antecedents and its perfect form and possibilities of development are thereby impaired. The process of development may go on until such time as some disturbing element, as excessive joy, fright or anger, or some of the zymotic diseases, come in contact with the disturbed vital energy, when it bursts forth into volcanic action and we see the manifestations of what we call acute diseases.

Sometimes this comes as the first outward and visible sign of a disturbed vital energy. It is analogous to the disturbance that takes place in waters, ponds, and reservoirs, when they suddenly begin to heave, seemingly without cause, and throw upward their pathogenetic formations, becoming exceedingly roily, to spend their efforts on this saprolytic action and so set in motion a clarifying process.

So it is with these manifestations in miasmatic conditions ; a blooming or explosion of these acute diseases is Nature's method of attempting to rid the system of these fundamental miasms that have been long buried. These manifestations offer to the homœopathic physician a unique opportunity to learn of the indicated remedy, because at the close of the acute manifestations Nature cries out most loudly and points the direction most clearly, because at this time symptoms are produced that are of inestimable value in the selection of the constitutional remedy. These diseased states—or disturbed states of the vital function—present very extensive and exceedingly variable external manifestations, and the homœopathic physician must devote much time to their study.

The vital force is always attempting to recover from diseased states. In the acute manifestations the vital functions are often restored to complete harmony by and through their own power, and it is noteworthy to observe the disappearance of symptoms in the reverse order of their appearance. This is well illustrated by the course of the appearance of symptoms in such manifestations as eruptive fevers—the rash appearing last is the first symptom to disappear ; the cough of measles, being the first symptom to appear, is the last to disappear. This order is always maintained in invasion and recession of symptoms when the vital force is able to establish complete restoration of normal vital functions.

Acute diseases may take on various forms. The assault may be so great as to destroy life in a short time. The vital force may be so overcome as to be unable to strive successfully against the combination of outward and inward assaults, and be completely destroyed. On the other hand, it may be able to overcome the disease conditions, without outside help, by crisis ; but when this happens, there is such a drain on the vital energy that it is a decided injury to the life-giving forces. Because of the sacrifice of fluids when crisis takes place, there is a lowering of the physical powers of the patient, and here again his very life is in danger.

When the vital force is not of itself able to make a

ʼmplete recovery, either due to a hidden miasm or an especially violent assault on the vital energy, the vital force often resorts to methods of bringing about a partial recovery. Thus the vital force pushes the invader out *en masse* by taking the inner trenches of the citadel and pushing the enemy to the outskirts of the country by establishing a semi-chronic skin manifestation ; or there may be establishment of a catarrhal disturbance on some one or more of the mucous surfaces, or the establishment of pus abscesses, with the expectation and hope of throwing out the enemy. Unfortunately the emptying of such abscesses may be into an organ or organs where complete expulsion from the body is not possible, as in pyothorax or pustular appendices.

Remedies will assist in these acute diseases and very, very often save the sacrifice of the crisis, and thereby the loss of physical power. It will always remain unknown how this power works in conjunction with the homœopathic remedy, to assist in conquering the assaults of the vital force, but that it does so and lowers very markedly the mortality rate in the acute diseases we know to be true. In acute diseases only is it ever possible for the vital force to rectify the conditions without assistance. In chronic conditions this can never be done. The homœopathic remedy assists in the cure because it represents a superior force ; no cure can take place unless a superior force is exhibited. The most potent force in the world of medicine is the potentized remedy, more potent by far than is the diseased condition.

Under a cure, the symptoms of a deranged vital function always disappear in the reverse order of their appearance. This is true in acute as well as chronic disturbances. Because this order is always maintained it is a vital point of observation in taking the case to note the sequence of symptoms in invasion, so that the physician can know of the progress of the case under the selected remedy. In very serious cases, when we are so anxious to know what improvement is taking place, we can be assured by watching the order of the disappearance of the symptoms. In this way we can learn the action of the remedy in its assistance to the vital force, and can give an accurate prognosis. This is equally true in acute or chronic states.

Too much stress cannot be laid upon the importance of the law of direction of cure of diseased states. Every physician should have this thoroughly ingrained into his consciousness. By cure we mean the complete eradication of diseased states and consequently the complete eradication of the symptoms, and a return to a condition of normal, vigorous health. The vital force must first be set in order by the indicated remedy, and the understanding of this great law of cure has proven of inestimable value in this process, in that we can know definitely whether we are proceeding in the manner that will lead to ultimate cure of the patient, or whether we are merely palliating or suppressing conditions.

IMPROVEMENT AND CURE COME FROM WITHIN OUTWARD. Just as no growth and development can take place from outside inward, so no hope of cure can be held that moves in a contrary direction. Growth and development and cure are centrifugal and never centripetal.

SYMPTOMS DISAPPEAR FROM ABOVE DOWNWARD ; COMPLAINTS GO FROM AN IMPORTANT ORGAN TO A LESS IMPORTANT ORGAN ; SYMPTOMS DISAPPEAR IN THE REVERSE ORDER OF THEIR APPEARANCE.

One of the best illustrations is the rheumatic fever manifestation. This is a case where the joints of the extremities are first attacked, next the joints nearer the body, and presently we find the heart involved. This is the natural order of the onset of the symptoms. Now if we relieve the symptoms appearing in the extremities, are we approaching a cure ? Consider the vital organs that are in danger, if they are not already attacked. But under the exhibition of the carefully selected homœopathic remedy the more important organs are the first to be freed (being the last organs to be attacked) and gradually the manifestations recede to the extremities, the first to be attacked.

It is absolutely necessary that these axioms be thoroughly grounded in our minds ; then it is a pleasure to feel the security that develops from our sure knowledge in the progress of any given case.

This pertains also to the artificial disease condition that we get from the drug proving. The onslaught of these symptoms is the same as in natural disease. They come on from below and move upward, or appear first in a superficial organ and then later move to a deeper organ. When a proving is wearing off, the symptoms recede in the reverse order, just as natural disease symptoms recede. This once more shows the relationship between the natural disease symptoms arising from a disturbed vital energy and the artificial disease symptoms as produced by a drug. This explains also the reason why the potentized drug is so effective in disease conditions ; the action of the remedy must follow the same cycle of action, under the same laws, as the natural action of the disturbed vital energy.

In chronic conditions this law is just as sure as in acute conditions, but in chronic conditions we are often faced with a seeming confusion. We have carefully taken the symptoms as reported by the patient, and have made our prescription. After a certain progress the patient comes to us with a new set of symptoms. Careful reference to the symptomatology shows no apparent relation to the present symptom-picture. Are we progressing in the right direction ? Is this a new condition that has arisen ? Let us proceed carefully. By cautious questioning we shall probably find that this is a return of old symptoms in the reverse order of appearance, and that it has been long covered up and forgotten because of the later unfolding of symptoms. Then as the later symptoms have disappeared, this older group has again come to the surface. Now we may know that we are proceeding in the proper direction. Right here great care must be taken not to mix the case. If the remedy is doing this work, let it proceed without interference, and the patient will lose these symptoms and a still older, more deeply buried group will presently come to the surface.

The necessity of constant study of the philosophy that underlies homœopathy becomes more and more apparent if we would be masters of our work ; and not only study, but a certain degree of patience to wait the course of events. However, if we can know that we are proceeding in the right direction, it gives us the patience and the courage to wait events, knowing that the prognosis is favourable and our work is effective.

To what do we attribute the growth and development of the individual ?

What is the direction of growth ?

What is health ?

What is disease ?

What do we mean by miasms or dyscrasias, and what is their effect on the development of the individual ?

How do we regard acute diseases ?

What conditions do we speak of as self-curative ?

How do we regard such conditions as semi-chronic or chronic skin manifestations, discharges, etc. ?

What is the order of cure ?

In taking a case, why do we consider the sequence of symptoms in their onset to be an important point ?

CHAPTER V

VITAL ENERGY IN ITS UNIVERSAL APPLICATION

THE vital energy is that force which animates each individual. While the vital energy is in the individual, that individual is said to have life, to be, to exist. Even as the individual is derived from—becomes—from the mating of two individuals, from the cell mating of which this vital force may be handed on with physical characteristics of the parents, so is the vital force itself derived from an infinite source, a storehouse of dynamic power, capable of developing and reproducing to an infinite degree in its manifestations, yet each individual partaking in greater or less degree of general vital characteristics common to all.

The vital force in the individual becomes therefore the ego, that most intimate spark of the individual which is in itself the essence of the individual, and which divides his individuality from all others, yet is his closest relationship to the universe. This closely relates him to all living creatures, yet he is identical with none ; it is at once his tie to all energy, all vitality, all life, and at the same time his insulation against the massed power of the whole.

Probably religion was the first expression of thought to formulate this vital concept of life. Many religions, through many ages, have expressed the thought we find in the Bible : " And the Lord God . . . breathed into his nostrils the breath of life ; and man became a living soul." " Before Abraham was, I AM." Religion accepts the concepts of infinite life on the spiritual plane, but has not attempted to apply it to all planes of existence ; science accepts it in part, one is tempted to say in fragments, but science has never correlated the whole, even on the material or intellectual planes.

Astronomy is a part of science ; mathematics is an essential component of astronomy. Astronomy and mathematics, viewed in the light of the whole vision of vital energy are essentially a partial proof of the omnipresence of vital energy as being the moving Energy, the activating Power, of the universe.

As Logic deals with " the principles governing the comparative and constructive faculties in the pursuit and use of truth ", let us apply this science to our theorem, and reason this through to its natural conclusions. Without this vital force there can be no life, no development. Since there is no static condition in nature, without a healthy normal development of the vital force we find a state of decay and death.

As homœopathic philosophers we do not concern ourselves at this time with the sociological aspects of this problem, although inferences from the foregoing statements may seem obvious ; it is our duty to consider these primarily as they relate to the physical, mental and spiritual well-being of our patients.

We have observed, in the study of the human race, that life is perpetuated under certain favourable conditions of mating. It is true that physical characteristics are handed on from parents to offspring, but that the parents actually give life to the child we may reasonably doubt. We may say with all assurance that under favourable circumstances life is handed on from the parents to the child, in more or less perfect vigour. Whence life comes we cannot say, but that it gives vigour in greater or less degree to the individual according to the heredity and environment we cannot doubt.

That life is continuous we know to be true ; there has been no age when all life has ceased, and we find this vital force, this energy, this dynamis, passed on in all forms and degrees of living creatures. History shows us that life has thus been manifest for so many centuries that we come by deductive reasoning to comprehend that life is infinite ; it is eternally going on and on.

Where there is vital force there is action, motion ; action is one interpretation, one manifestation, of vital force. We speak of the inanimate as dead, yet with death there is always decay. We think of the earth and other plants as dead, yet they are in continual motion, according to their regular and defined direction through the universe, which has been observed and recorded by man. We may reason, therefore, that since these great bodies have regular motion and direction, they are impelled by some force, some energy, which although it may not be what we have come to call vital energy, is in degree closely related to it.

If therefore this force, this energy, actuates or permeates all forms and degrees of life from the most humble and inconspicuous to the very planets, we may reasonably assume that vital force is the most fundamental of all conditions of the universe, and that the laws governing the vital force in the individual are correlated with the laws which govern all vital force, all forms of energy, wherever or however expressed.

If we have no motion, no action, no direction, without vital energy, it must be this energy which is responsible for all growth and all development in all spheres of existence.

Like all laws, the laws governing vital force may be infringed to some degree. The privilege granted to human life is the right of choice, and this right of choice implies degrees of choice. The planets, being set in their courses, have no right of choice and move always according to law. Human beings we know to exercise the right of choice, and herein is our province as physicians, for in making the choice, which is often a choice against natural laws, we find the vigour of the vital force abated and a retrograde action of the body, mind, or spirit sets in. As we have pointed out before, vital force in its perfection means growth and development ; since there is no condition of standing still in nature, an infringement of natural laws means decay and death. The degree of the infringement, either in an individual or in his predecessors, determines the degree of decay and its speed.

Since human beings as individuals have the right of choice, even in the face of the operation of the natural laws governing the vital energy, they have also been given those circumstances and conditions surrounding them which tend toward, (1) a correct choice (direction), and (2) aids to correct the mistakes already made and to regain the normal balance. Both these conditions are found in three spheres, the physical, the mental, and the spiritual.

On the spiritual plane we find those aids which tend toward correct choice and aids to regain a lost balance in the form of religious convictions and beliefs, all those aids which foster the growth and development of the spiritual life of man. On the mental plane we find instruction of various kinds which tends to development of the mental faculties and all those things which go toward an honest comprehension of the individual toward himself and his relationship to others and toward all life ; in other words, those things which foster sanity. On the physical plane we find those things which tend to keep us healthy in body, such as suitable foods and those things which we can adapt for better housing, cleanliness, sanitation, and many other things. We find on this plane, too, many substances closely allied to foods which have within them a vital energy capable of being raised by potentization from the purely physical plane to that of the mental or even spiritual. This is most decidedly the study of the homœopathic physician, for in these substances we find the most similar remedies for the conditions of the ills of man.

These substances themselves are derived from three kingdoms, mineral, vegetable, and animal. We cannot definitely say that the mineral substances in themselves possess vital energy, but they are fragments of that which composes the planet, earth, and that planet either possesses some form of vital energy in itself or is susceptible to being activated by vital energy to such an extent that it performs its appointed movements according to the law ; and we can use these minerals, by proper preparation, in the form of vital energy, not to perpetuate life but to influence it on all three planes of body, mind, and spirit, that the vital energy of the individual may be thereby guarded against decay and death.

We recognize the presence of vital energy in vegetable growth, for it is evidenced in growth and movement in the plant, according to the natural law of development, from within outward ; the plant develops from the seed according to the physical characteristics of the parents, and again under favourable circumstances passes on this spark of vital energy in its own fertility. Not only do we know that vegetable growth has this manifestation of vital energy, but it has been observed that the mysterious vital force, beyond our comprehension, which controls by law the planets in their courses and influences the winds and tides, influences the manner and periods of growth of the individual plant, thus again tying what we know to be a manifestation of life to the universal energy.

The vegetable kingdom has probably served man in disease conditions longer than either the animal or the mineral kingdom. In the homœopathic method of preparing drugs for medication, by releasing the energy therein through potentization, we have found that from this source again which we regard as material we can influence disorder on the three planes of body, mind, and spirit.

We comprehend most easily the animation, the presence of vital energy, in the animal kingdom, and medicine has long sought cure through the medium of substances derived from this source. That these substances have a tremendous power we know to be true. Homœopathy, however, in distinction from ordinary medicine, believes that there, too, the release of power from the minimum of substance through potentization is that which will most quickly and accurately influence the disordered vital force of man on all three planes.

We believe that vital energy as we comprehend it is not a mass power, but an infinite number of egocentric sparks. We believe also that material substance, mass power, in medication, would completely overwhelm the individual vital energy to complete annihilation or would subvert it to eventual decay and death. We believe that the mathematical law of quantity extends through all nature, and applies to all vital energy in whatever form, and that if this is so, it is peculiarly applicable when we are dealing with that infinitely delicate balance of vital force in the individual.

Let us look at this law of mathematics with that thought in mind : THE QUANTITY OF ACTION NECESSARY TO EFFECT ANY CHANGE IN NATURE IS THE LEAST POSSIBLE ; and, as Fincke added : THE DECISIVE AMOUNT IS ALWAYS A MINIMUM, AN INFINITESIMAL.

If vital energy is the fundamental power, the motivating factor of the universe, balance must be one expression of the law. If the very planets are kept in their place through the influence of vital energy, this must be an infinitely delicate balance. We see the effects of balance all through nature and natural expressions and therefore we realize that balance, power, is one manifestation of the law. Since the earth upon which we live is so delicately poised that it holds its regular position and movements without deviation, according to law, anything upon the earth which lives or is subject to the influence of vital energy must therefore in some degree be susceptible to balance. We recognize more susceptibility to the manifestations and interplay of vital energy and balance in the individuals of the human race than in any other form of existence, since we so often see the effects of the imbalance of the individual. This is doubtless due to the influence of his power of choice, which often influences his own dynamis and the dynamis of those with whom he comes in contact. In other words, his very existence is an expression of vital energy, but he is also exposed to the influence of the vital energy of others and the interplay of vital energy and balance from many sources may imperil his own balance. The resultant lack of balance in his own vital energy is disorder that manifests itself in a train of symptoms of dis-ease.

Mathematics is the science which treats of the measuring of quantities and the ascertainment of their properties and relations ; this is an exact science. It is a part of the study of astronomy, among other natural studies, and it must be applicable in all spheres where any concept of measurement or relationship exists. Balance is the state of perfect relation- ship, the result of perfect computation, and the desired goal of all mathematics. We might say that mathematics in its highest form is the perception of balance in its highest degree. Thus we realize that the laws that apply to mathematics must be equally applicable to every condition where balance is a factor.

Lack of balance in the individual may be engendered by the interplay of forces resulting from his privilege of choice, from the interplay of forces engendered by others and over which he has little or no control, or by the released power of an infinitesimal amount of almost any substance, animal vegetable, or mineral, which has in itself the susceptibility of permeation or activation of vital energy.   Here we see the applicability of the mathematical law. *The quantity of action* (the actual quantity of substance susceptible to action) *necessary to effect any change in nature* (necessary to affect the balance of any living thing or the relationship between any living thing and circumstances) *is the least possible.   The decisive amount is always a minimum, an infinitesimal.*

All the elements, and all forms of matter, are capable of being moved, activated, by vital energy, although they may not themselves possess this energy within themselves.   All the elements and all forms of matter possess the possibility of divisibility to an almost infinite degree.   The greater the mass (quantity) of elements or matter, the more inert they become.   Thus, massed iron becomes useful to man as iron or steel rails, bridges, utensils, or other material objects. Iron in a divided state enters into the human physical body as a component part of that which is activated by the vital energy, and as a part of the physical body the vital energy plays through it.   Iron, even when massed and inert, has the power of attracting vital energy in the form of electricity, but iron in mass formation is not capable of balance and direction within itself to the degree that is possible when its divisibility is greater.

It is a question whether matter itself, which we call at times inert, does not manifest active properties ; in other words, is possessed by activity and motion.   This has been demonstrated in Madame Curie's investigations of radioactive substances, and again in the far-reaching discoveries of Languin in his demonstration of the activity within the atom of the physical cells.

The greater the divisibility of elements or matter, the more they exhibit the possibility of permeability by the vital energy ; the energy being not dependent upon the mass, but on the play or balance between the positive and negative poles of the atom.

Vital force is capable of three forms of action : motion, direction, and balance.   These manifestations of energy are an integral part of any exhibition of vital energy.   Growth and development are directed motion, and in the degree of their perfection do we find the manifestation of balance.

What do we mean by vital energy ?

What is the influence of energy on growth and development ?

What is the effect of potentization on material substances ?

How is the energy inherent in plants released for their use in remedies ?

State the mathematical law of least action.

How does the law of least action apply to the administration of homœopathic potentized remedies ?

What influence has divisibility upon matter ?

What three forms of action has vital force ?

CHAPTER VI

HOMŒOPATHY AND THE FUNDAMENTAL LAWS

AMONG the followers of Hahnemann we often hear the statement that homœopathy is fundamental; that it is scientific; that it is based on natural law. Let us grant, for the sake of argument, that this is true; the natural corollary of this statement is that these laws must be active in all realms of fundamental science, i.e. that in those sciences that deal with the established laws of the universe the same natural laws must be active. It is self-evident that natural laws must work, not in contradiction to each other, but in sympathy and co-operation; these laws are fixed and immutable. That which sets the planet in its orbit so regulates the other planets that they obey the same laws; their difference lies not in the governing laws but in time, distance and circumstance, which is again ruled by law. If the planets moved at random lawlessly, the result would be chaos.

So, too, if one realm of the universe was moved by fundamental laws which had no application or relation to other realms of the universe, the result must be chaos. If one science is seemingly governed by laws which are contradictory to those of another science, one must be lawless, not a science, or not science but chaos would be the result.

IF HOMŒOPATHY IS A FUNDAMENTAL SCIENCE, OR A PART OF A FUNDAMENTAL SCIENCE, AS WE BELIEVE, IT MUST WORK IN HARMONY WITH ALL THE NATURAL REALMS, AND THE LAWS WHICH APPLY TO THOSE REALMS MUST APPLY ALSO, IN SOME DEGREE AND RELATIONSHIP, TO HOMŒOPATHY.

In spite of the years that have been devoted to the study of homœopathy, with their accumulated data, we glimpse but dimly the possibilities of these conclusions. When we realize the confusion that man has caused in his individual life, in every sphere, it is little wonder that he has misunderstood the natural powers and resources, and has failed to make use of natural laws. It is not strange, then, that medicine, among many other phases of our modern life, is but a series of experimental gropings without form or order.

The glimpse at our present state of social confusion cannot excuse our refusal to substantiate our claim that homœopathy is based on natural laws. Let us consider the place homœopathy must hold if our contentions be true. If homœopathy is founded upon fundamental laws, what are some of those laws ? Our ignorance permits us to register but a few, but inevitably the time will come, if we keep a clear vision, when we will be able to add more to our burden of proof.

Let us look at the first formulated and recognized law of homœopathy, SIMILIA SIMILIBUS CURENTUR. Whence came this law ? It was simply an intelligent observation of our natural resources, those in their closest proximity to our daily lives, in the vegetable kingdom, and their relation to disturbed and disordered conditions arising in mankind himself. It was found that the ills of individual man could be successfully treated thus ; first doubtless these substances were found in the vegetable kingdom, later in the mineral and animal kingdom also. Still later came the knowledge that this was not by chance, an occasional means of cure, but that by law these substances acted in an ordered and orderly manner under certain definite conditions and circumstances.

This recognition of law underlying cure is of ancient origin ; no one knows when the first recognition of this law crept into use, but ancient Hindu manuscripts recorded its application. Certainly Aristotle recognized it, and Hippocrates sensed the possibilities of this law and applied it in some recorded cases. From time to time all through medical history this hypothesis was enunciated or demonstrated in greater or less degree. Hahnemann later demonstrated this law to be universal and not an occasional circumstance. He called the science and art of healing which naturally followed, *homœopathy*, but the thought was not a new one ; it was age-old before a science of healing was based solely on this law.

In other words, in even the embryonic stages of homœopathy it was found that *law governed*. Gradual experimentation widened the possibilities of application of these laws ; no amount of experimentation extended the laws themselves. All that experimentation could do was to enlighten our minds regarding the scope of the law.

A law is a fundamental fact ; because we do not recognize a law does not mean that the law does not exist. Even to man-made laws, which in their essence are not laws in the true sense but rules laid down by man for man, it is recognized that ignorance of the law is no excuse.

As observation became focused upon the unfolding of the law of cure, other regularities in reaction were discovered, and a second law of cure, this time pertaining to the direction of cure, was formulated. This was : CURE TAKES PLACE FROM ABOVE DOWNWARD, FROM WITHIN OUTWARD, FROM AN IMPORTANT ORGAN TO A LESS IMPORTANT ORGAN ; SYMPTOMS DISAPPEAR IN THE REVERSE ORDER OF THEIR APPEARANCE, THE FIRST TO APPEAR BEING THE LAST TO DISAPPEAR.

Simple disappearance of symptoms is by no means cure ; symptoms often have periods of recurrence, but no true cure has ever been observed that did not follow the law of direction.

Another law, equally applicable throughout the universe, is that of mutual action : ACTION AND REACTION ARE EQUAL AND OPPOSITE.

To some of us who have thoughtfully considered these things they seem so self-evident that it would be almost unnecessary to speak of them were it not for the purpose of urging you to observe the lawfulness of homœopathy, and to prove our claim of the fundamental lawfulness of this true science of healing. Let us look at a law which follows naturally the law of mutual action.

This is the law designated as the *law of least action*, which was formulated by Maupertius, the French mathematician. To us as homœopathic physicians and students it may be known as the law of quantity and dose : THE QUANTITY OF ACTION NECESSARY TO EFFECT ANY CHANGE IN NATURE IS THE LEAST POSSIBLE ; THE DECISIVE AMOUNT IS ALWAYS A MINIMUM, AN INFINITESIMAL.

Health is a matter of perfect equilibrium, perfect balance ; trifling circumstances may sway it, and even as seemingly trifling circumstances may sway it, so may it be balanced by the least possible in medication, which may, in conditions of perfect health, cause the same loss of balance, or a *corresponding* loss of equilibrium.

Another law of quantity to be considered here is : THE QUANTITY OF THE DRUG REQUIRED IS IN INVERSE RATIO TO THE SIMILARITY.   In other words, the greater the similarity of the drug symptoms to those of the patient, the less quantity will be required, for the greater will be the state of susceptibility of the patient.

A corollary to the law of quantity is: THE QUALITY OF THE ACTION OF A HOMŒOPATHIC REMEDY IS DETERMINED BY ITS QUANTITY, IN INVERSE RATIO.   Again this is a problem of the susceptibility of the patient and the similarity of the drug ; the laws of quality and quantity go hand in hand.

Biology gives us this law : FUNCTION CREATES AND DEVELOPS THE ORGAN.   It has been observed in the study of homœopathy that functional symptoms are produced by the vital force in exact proportion to the profundity of the disturbance.   Often, however, when pathological changes occur the symptomatic picture changes greatly in that functional symptoms do not manifest themselves in as great a degree ; the disease condition has struck deeper and manifests itself less on the surface.   Following the biological law, therefore, homœopathy postulates the law of symptom development : FUNCTIONAL SYMPTOMS PRECEDE STRUCTURAL CHANGES.

Now the law of use governing the homœopathic remedy must therefore be : THE DOSE AND QUANTITY THAT WILL THOROUGHLY PERMEATE THE ORGANISM AND MAKE ITS ESSENTIAL IMPRESS UPON THE VITAL FORCE IS THAT WHICH WILL AFFECT THE FUNCTIONAL SPHERE OF THE INDIVIDUAL.

We say : " This must therefore be " ; if we reason logically, and have observed carefully, keeping our line of reasoning along the lines of laws already formulated and proven sound, we can do no less than believe that this is a truly fundamental law.

For many years daily practice has proven the value of

the law of repetition of the dose : NEVER REPEAT YOUR REMEDY SO LONG AS IT CONTINUES TO ACT. This governs the administration of remedies to individuals in states of disease ; let us look at the law that must govern the production of symptoms by artificial means, i.e. drug provings, by which we get our guidance for the administration of drugs to the sick. The object of proving drugs is the production of artificial diseases that we may observe the symptoms and apply the substances so proven in like states of natural disturbance. The law governing this must be closely allied to the law of administration in states of disease, or else our case is not logical. We find this law : NEVER REPEAT THE DOSE IN A PROVING WHILE SYMPTOMS ARE MANIFEST FROM THE DOSE ALREADY TAKEN.

Again granting that homœopathy is allied to all nature, we must concede that orbits or cycles of action are a fundamental part of natural manifestations. So also we find that the homœopathic remedies have cycles of development and recession. If the natural cycle of symptom development is interfered with, we gain no knowledge of the true nature of the substance being proved ; at best we can get but a distorted comprehension of its nature when there is any interference. Continuing to administer repeatedly a remedy while it is producing disease symptoms in a prover would make chaos out of a normal cycle of disease symptoms which have been in process of development. This is simply the result of logical reasoning.

Examining still further into laws governing the production of artificial disease states, we find there are laws governing the various states or types of substances which we desire to prove. As yet we may find these laws crudely phrased, but they follow closely the law of mutual action, the law of least action, and the laws of quantity and quality.

I.   ANY DRUG WHICH IN ITS NATURAL STATE AFFECTS THE VITAL ENERGY BUT LITTLE WILL DEVELOP A PROVING *only* IN A HIGH POTENCY.

2.   ANY DRUG WHICH IN ITS NATURAL STATE DISTURBS THE VITAL ENERGY TO *functional* MANIFESTATIONS ONLY *may* BE PROVEN IN A CRUDE FORM.

3.   ANY DRUG WHICH IN ITS NATURAL STATE DISTURBS

THE VITAL ENERGY TO DESTRUCTIVE MANIFESTATIONS SHOULD BE PROVEN *only* IN A POTENTIATED FORM.

It has been demonstrated that planetary movements have a definite relationship to life. The power of the moon over the tides is an ancient and constant observation. The relationship of the earth and the sun offers an irrefutable argument in favour of the correlation of the planetary influences. The influence of the phases of the moon on some mental conditions and nervous complaints has been noted from the earliest times. For instance, the appellation *lunacy* designated a mental disturbance definitely related to moon phases ; epileptic conditions also have shown some response to the cycles of the moon. In other words, through these abnormal conditions of mental and nervous disturbance we have perceived dimly from time to time the outlines of a great truth.

That cyclic manifestations have been demonstrated in other fields than medicine is easily seen from the most cursory glance at the science of astronomy. In its earlier stages astronomy suffered from the same blind groping, ignorance and superstition that has hampered the intelligent observation of all natural phenomena ; nevertheless, it has emerged as a true science of mathematical exactness. It is still true that the deductions from the most careful measurements and computations vary between different schools, yet it is the most closely measurable of all the sciences to-day.

Let us quote from *The Concise Knowledge of Astronomy : History*, by Agnes M. Clerke, pages 12, 13 :

The subjection of the moon to known law was completed by the dispersal of the mystery surrounding a slight, continuous acceleration of her orbital velocity detected by Halley in 1693. It had been in progress since the earliest recorded eclipse in 721 B.C., if not longer ; there was no sign of its cessation or reversal, and the grave question arose: Was the principle of universal attraction elsewhere unreservedly obeyed, here fatally complicated by the action of a resisting medium involving the eventual collapse of the earth-moon system ? Laplace gave the answer in 1787 by proving the observed quickening of pace to be a necessary and simple consequence of a secular diminution in the ellipticity of the earth's orbit. This, however, will not go on forever in the same direction ; after many ages the tide of change will turn, and a complete restoration to *status quo ante* will ensue. . . . Ruinous disturbances were shown to be excluded by the overwhelming disparity of mass between the central body and its attendants, no less than by the regularity and harmony of their movements and distribution. Thus only slight oscillatory changes can occur. Millions of years will elapse without producing any fundamental alteration. The machine is so beautifully adjusted as to right itself automatically through the mutual action of its various parts. And it is the force which perturbs that eventually restores.

Let us repeat the last lines of this quotation in the light of our observation into the relation of homœopathy and the fundamental laws : *The machine is so beautifully adjusted as to right itself automatically through the mutual action of its various parts.* AND IT IS THE FORCE WHICH PERTURBS THAT EVENTUALLY RESTORES.

This last observation, acknowledged by the most exact of all sciences and a deduction from observation of the most observable of all cyclic phenomena, is equally pertinent to homœopathy and our belief in the lawful flow of vital energy. This deduction, so fundamental that it might well be called a law, is closely allied to that law of mathematics : *The quantity of action necessary to effect any change in nature is the least possible.*

These are but a few of the laws which we, in our ignorance, have assembled from the vast resources at our command to demonstrate that homœopathy is governed by laws that are universal, and that homœopathy, therefore, is a part of the fundamental lawfulness and orderliness of the universe. If we can apply a known law of biology, a known law of mathematics, and a known and accepted deduction of astronomy, we can as surely apply the tested laws of any other sphere of universal activity.

At some future time we will be able to formulate definitely those laws which govern the vital force and its action in the human economy. This vital energy, which is the sun of our individual human economy, has a distinct relationship to universal vital energy. It is vital energy in the individual which offers homœopathy its scientific demonstration of healing. Of this mystery we now comprehend but this : The state of the disordered vital energy is that state in which homœopathy offers the greatest hope of regaining the lost balance of power in each individual, and that not by coercion of the vital force, but by so stimulating it that the equilibrium is restored by the same force that disturbed it ; that the vital energy in itself is capable of disturbance and of self-restoration under the proper circumstances. We have used the laws of homœopathy half blindly, as it were, yet we recognize their tremendous significance and their possibilities; we have observed their action in countless cases of human misery.

Let us be alert to observe and accurate to correlate the plain facts before us, that we may recognize, formulate and work in accord with the fundamental laws that govern homœopathy and all nature.

HOMŒOPATHIC LAWS

OF CURE :

Similia similibus curentur.

Cure takes place from above downward, from within outward, from the more important to the less important organ, and in the reverse order of the onset of the symptoms.

OF ACTION :

Action and reaction are equal and opposite.

OF QUANTITY AND DOSE :

The quantity of the drug required is in inverse ratio to the similarity.

OF QUANTITY :

The quantity of action necessary to effect any change in Nature is the least possible. The decisive amount is always a minimum, an infinitesimal.

OF QUALITY :

The quality of the action of a homœopathic remedy is determined by its quantity, in inverse ratio.

OF USE :

The dose and quantity that will thoroughly permeate the organism and make its essential impress upon the vital force is that which will affect the functional sphere of the individual.

OF BIOLOGICAL DEVELOPMENT :

Function creates and develops the organ.

OF DISEASE DEVELOPMENT :

Functional symptoms are produced by the vital force in exact proportion to the profundity of the disturbance. Functional symptoms precede structural changes.

OF PROVING :

1. Any drug which in its natural state affects the vital energy but little will develop a proving only in a high potency.
2. Any drug which in its natural state disturbs the vital energy to functional manifestations only *may* be proven in a crude form.
3. Any drug which in its natural state disturbs the vital energy to destructive manifestations should be proven only in a potentiated form.

OF REPETITION (for Provings) :

Never repeat the dose while symptoms are manifest from the dose already taken.

OF REPETITION (for Cure) :

Never repeat your remedy so long as it continues to act

CHAPTER VII

OUR REMEDIES : WHY THEY ACT

IN our thesis that homœopathy is fundamental, that it is scientific and that it is based on natural law, we have quoted findings from other branches of pure science that have been so uniform and constant as to definitely point the way toward underlying laws. These, to recapitulate briefly, were from astronomy, mathematics and biology, and have been compared with the closely similar findings of the action of drugs and their application (1) in states of health to produce, artificially, conditions simulating disease, or (2) to restore diseased states to the normal balance of health.

Let us consider once more some of our deductions set forth in former chapters on " Vital Energy ", and particularly in that chapter on " Vital Energy in its Universal Application ". That we may have it before us for examination in comparing our deductions from other branches of scientific investigation with our study of the natural laws underlying the principles adapted for use in the science of healing known as homœopathy, we shall quote from these chapters :

These substances (capable of being raised by potentization) are derived from three kingdoms, mineral, vegetable and animal. We cannot definitely say that the mineral substances in themselves possess vital energy, but they are fragments of that which composes the planet, Earth, and that planet either possesses some form of vital energy in itself or is susceptible to being activated by vital energy to such an extent that it performs its appointed movements according to the law ; and we can use these minerals, by proper preparation, in the form of vital energy, not to perpetuate life but to influence it on all three planes of body, mind and spirit, that the vital energy of the individual may be thereby guarded against decay and death. . . .

We recognize the presence of vital energy in vegetable growth, for it is evidenced in growth and development on the plant, according to the natural law of development. . . .

We comprehend most easily the animation, the presence of vital energy, in the animal kingdom. . . .

It is quite within the province of the homœopathic physician, especially if he believes that homœopathy is based on the fundamental principles underlying all elemental construction and development, to attempt to understand something of the basis of the elements with which he has to deal, both in states of sickness and in health. This implies a knowledge of drugs, not only their action but their derivation, and this not in superficial terms, but in terms of basic derivation and inter-relation with universal construction. This deals with physics in a very definite way, and in a much deeper, more constructive and significant way than we usually consider.

In his little book, *Science and the New Civilization*, Millikan gives us some valuable hints in his chapter on " Available Energy "   His statement in this chapter is that :

All knowledge that helps towards an understanding of the nature of the universe of which we are a part is useful, for we need very much more of it than we now have, or shall have for centuries to come, to enable us to direct our energies towards wise, effective living instead of wasting them on beating tom-toms, inventing perpetual motion machines, or chasing either physical or social rainbows.

If it be wise for the average person to direct their energies toward an understanding of things about them, how much more is it the province of him who is entrusted with the care of others through the use of drugs, built up and potentized out of the elements !

Let us consider further some of Dr. Millikan's statements in this chapter, and their bearing on our specialty.

It is interesting and a very important fact from the practical viewpoint, too, that more than ninety-five per cent. of this universe, so far as we can now see, is made up of a very few elements.

First. The spectroscopy of the heavens shows the enormous prevalence everywhere of hydrogen, but hydrogen is merely the primordial positive and negative electrons tied together, or in process of being so tied.

Second. The spectroscopy of the heavens also shows that helium is an exceptionally abundant, and a widely distributed element, even though, because of its lightness and inability to combine with anything, even with itself, the earth has not retained much of it. Significant is it, however, that the alpha particle given off by all the heavy radioactive elements is nothing but helium, so that it must have a certain prevalence even on earth in the structure of the heavier elements.

Third. Dr. I. S. Bowen, at the California Institute, solved, with consummate skill, the half-century-old riddle of "nebulium", and has shown that the substance, abundant throughout the heavens, giving rise to these mysterious spectral lines, is mainly oxygen and nitrogen. But oxygen alone constitutes 55 per cent. of the earth's crust, and about the same proportion of meteorites. Oxygen and nitrogen, then, which for our present purpose will be treated as one element, since they have nearly the same atomic weight and will be henceforth listed under the name of the stronger brother, constitute the third extraordinarily abundant element and it is to be noted that there are no abundant elements at all between helium and oxygen. Carbon has a certain minor prevalence, but because of its nearness in atomic weight to nitrogen and oxygen it may here be treated as merely a feeble satellite to oxygen.

Fourth. Ninety-five per cent. of the weight of all meteorites consists of oxygen (54 per cent.), magnesium (13 per cent.), silicon (15 per cent.) and iron (13 per cent.), while 76 per cent. of the earth's crust is composed of the three elements, oxygen (55 per cent.), silicon (16 per cent.), and aluminium (5 per cent.), no other element rising over 2 per cent. Iron constitutes 1·5 per cent. of the crust, but it is supposed to be very largely represented in the interior. Because of the closeness of their atomic weights, magnesium, aluminium and silicon (24, 27, 28) may, for our present purpose, be regarded as a single element and given the name of the strongest brother, silicon. There are then no abundant elements whatever between oxygen and silicon, nor between silicon and iron (atomic weight 56), and from an *engineering standpoint the universe may be said to be made up of the* primordial positive and negative electrons, and of four *elements built out of them, namely, helium, oxygen, silicon and iron.*

. . . Mankind, if he is here a billion years hence, will be satisfying his main needs, as he satisfies them now, with the four elements, hydrogen, oxygen, silicon and iron, *i.e.* with water, air, earth and Fe, where the last symbol stands for iron rather than for fire, which was the fourth constituent of the world of the ancients.

To comprehend the action of our remedies it is well to look somewhat to the sources from which our remedies are derived and to weigh their possible activity in their natural state.

We regard the sources of drugs as lying in three distinct groups—animal, vegetable, and mineral ; or we may make two classifications and say *living* and *non-living*.

Sir J. C. Bose, in his *Plant Autographs and Their Revelations*, writes :

Do not the two sets of records of the living and non-living tell us of some property of matter common and persistent ? Do they not show us that the same kind of molecular upset on stimulation occurs on both the inorganic and the living—that the physiological is closely connected with the physical—that there is no abrupt break, but a uniform march of law ? The dust particle and the earth, the plant and the animal, are all sensitive. Thus, with an enlarged cosmic sense, we may regard the million orbs that thread their path through space, as something akin to organisms, having a definite history of their past and an evolutionary progress for their future.

And again :

In pursuing investigations on the border region of physics and physiology, I was amazed to find boundary lines vanishing and points of contact emerge between the realms of the Living and Non-living. Metals are found to respond to stimuli ; they are subject to fatigue, stimulated by certain drugs and " killed " by poisons.

For the purpose of convenience, however, we may divide drugs or substances from which homœopathic medications are prepared, into the three classes of animal, vegetable, and mineral (or elements).

We expect to find the highest form of living activity in animals. We have been taught to expect strong reaction to the various forms of defence of individual species of animal life. Thus, we find the venom of snakes has a deep action on other forms of animal life. We deduce that even when venom is prepared in minute doses, it will also have a strong

reaction on animal life. Sir J. C. Bose has verified this in
his experiments with the action of cobra venom (Naja) on
animals and plants. He found that in doses of 0·5 c.c. of
solution of venom, one part in a thousand, when injected into
the vein of a fish the heart stopped beating in twelve minutes.
This action was automatically recorded on delicate instruments. The same experiment was next applied to the plant,
a solution of one per cent. being used. A great depression
was first recorded, then the pulse-beat came to a permanent
stop, then came wilting and decomposition.

It is hardly necessary to go into the data available for
further proofs of the activity of snake venoms ; our homœopathic provings preceded by many years the acknowledgment
of the allopathic school that venoms in minute doses were
exceedingly efficacious in many serious conditions, especially
those showing great derangement of the vascular and nervous
systems.

That forms of defence, such as spider venoms, sepia, stings
of bees and insects, and many other natural weapons, have
been found effective in causing and treating bodily discomforts may not be denied by those who have observed
their action.

Thus we may pass on to a consideration of plant life as a
source from which we may expect to derive useful remedies.
We expect, and find, great reaction from all those growths
which manifest, in their natural states, the power of protec-
tion through defence by poisonous properties.   Thus we find
all members of the Rhus family exceedingly active, both in
their crude state and in potentized form, affecting strongly
the human organism in countless ways.

The list of plants that strongly affect the human organism
ranges through all forms, from the forms that approach the
animal development in their power of capturing and devour-
ing insects, such as the Drosera and Sarracenia purpurea, to
the lowliest and hardiest growths, such as Sticta pulmonaria,
and is almost endless.   To do more than glance at the long
list of possibilities that open to the homœopathic physician
through this source would be a task far too long for one
chapter.   We may take ourselves at once to the observation
of those substances that may be most truly said to be

non-living, yet which must enter largely into the composition of the living, and that encompass us.

Even more deeply acting than the venoms, we find the mineral and chemical elements. Plant life, through its power of simplifying these substances readily, form the closest relationship to the mineral kingdom, for here the elements are often absorbed and made available for ingestion into the animal, directly or in new combinations that render them even more active. Thus we see the reasons for *Pulsatilla's* strong action on the human economy. Dr. Underhill tells us that *Pulsatilla* is one of the most effective chemical laboratories known, assimilating the mineral content and elements in the soil and rebuilding it into a most deep-acting and complicated influence upon the human organism.

The most cursory glance at the chemical elements of our most common plant remedies must reveal how deeply bound these are to the chemical elements of light weight—far below the atomic weight of those known to be radioactive—and these may be classed as those written of by Millikan (to quote again from the same source we have quoted above) :

. . . *For the great majority of the elements, such as constitute the bulk of our world, are in their state of maximum stability already.* They have no energy to give up in the disintegrating process. They can only be broken apart by working upon them, or by supplying energy to them. Man can probably learn to disintegrate them, but he will always do it " by the sweat of his brow ".

But having thus disposed of the process of atomic disintegration, and found it completely wanting as a source of available energy, since the radioactive elements are necessarily negligible in quantity, let us next see what there is to be learned about the process of *atom-building* as a source of energy. . . .

Millikan goes on :

. . . the recent experimental work on cosmic rays, have just thrown a flood of light on the process going on in this universe in which we live. For first Dr. Cameron and I have recently found three definite cosmic ray bands, or frequencies, of penetrating powers, or ray-energies, respectively, about twelve, fifty and one hundred times the maximum possible energies that are, or can be, obtained from any radioactive, that is, any disintegrating, process. The highest frequency band has so enormous a penetrating power that it passes through more than 200 feet of water or eighteen feet of lead before becoming completely absorbed, while two or three inches of lead absorbs the hardest gamma rays. This discovery of a banded structure in cosmic rays shows that these rays are not produced, as are X-rays, by the impact upon the atoms of matter of electrons that have acquired large velocities by falling through powerful electric fields, as we earlier suggested—the fields necessary to produce frequencies as high as those of the highest observed cosmic rays are equivalent to 216,000,000 volts—but that *they are rather produced by definite and continually recurring atomic transformations involving very much greater energy-chances than any occurring in radioactive processes.*

Taking Einstein's equation and Aston's curve as a guide there are no possible atomic transformations capable of yielding rays of the enormous penetrating power observed by us, except those corresponding to the building up or creation of the abundant elements like helium, oxygen, silicon, and iron out of hydrogen, or possibly in the case of the last two elements out of helium. . . . We have arrived at pretty definite evidence that *the observed cosmic rays are the signals broadcast throughout the heavens of the births of the common elements out of positive and negative electrons.*

Thus we find that in the birth of, say, two of our common earth elements, iron and silicon, we find tremendous powers liberated in the heavens. (For convenience Millikan in this article speaks of magnesium and aluminium as coincident with silicon, because of their close atomic weights.) We all know their effectiveness when energy is released by long trituration and powerful succussion. Chemical analysis of some of our common plant remedies reveals the presence of one or more of these common earth elements, assimilated, broken into a form that supplies life-energy to the plant. We find in a cursory examination of *Lycopodium clavatum* that it contains aluminium. Consider what this element, that has a powerful effect upon animal tissue and animal energy when its powers are released by reducing it to the form of the homœopathic potency—consider, I say, its profound effect after its assimilation by the plant, its energies there partially released for effective reaction, and that in turn undergoing a further breaking up and disintegration by the processes of trituration and potentization.

The history of the *Lycopodiaceæ* may be of still further interest in giving us the reason for its effectiveness. Among the old forms of life—those forms which have existed longest upon the earth—we find the mosses, and of these this family is a hardy member. It is probably one of the oldest living forms of earthy plant life (that is, dependent both upon soil and water). It has persisted past all changes in circumstances and conditions, and probably has changed its form less to meet changing conditions than almost any other form of life except possibly the *Equisetum*, another of the early surviving forms. This tenacity of life, adapting itself to circumstances without conforming, bespeaks a tenacity of energy that, when released, must powerfully effect that which it touches.

Equisetum hymenale contains silicon (in the form of oxide) and magnesium ; in analysis the amount of silicon may run from 7·5 per cent. to 41·2 per cent. If at their birth these elements register such tremendous energy as the cosmic waves reveal, what effectiveness must we expect when it has been assimilated, broken down, first in plant life and then by trituration and potentization even in minute quantities ?

When animal, vegetable or mineral substances are potentized they are rendered more potent because of the breaking up, disintegration of thin atomic relationships, that place them in a form where they act directly upon the dynamic force of the individual. That is, in their disintegration their energy is liberated by releasing the radioactive power. Through the radioactivity exerting itself upon the vital energy of the individual the potency is made effective.

Thus we are forced to recognize different forms of energy —the discharge of different energies or rays—from what we have considered as inanimate metals and elements. We find that they respond energetically in much the same way as plants and animals ; not alone in their simple states do we find this response, but again and again as they are assimilated, broken down and rebuilt in different forms of life, from the simple assimilation and complicated rebuilding of the plant to the profound reaction on all living substance when they are in potentized form.

We recognize that elements having high atomic weights are radioactive; they give off, spontaneously, rays of different velocity and penetrating power, and in their radioactivity, their dissemination of energy, they are themselves changed. Einstein expresses this change when he says : " The change of mass equals the change of energy. As they vary energy vanishes with the mass and so they are equal."

Mass, in this sense, does not mean bulk, as we commonly think of it. It is rather the sum total of that which gives off energy, or is capable of giving off energy, and of which energy in some form is a part. As in mathematics, that which remains after subtraction is not as great as before. One cannot go on subtracting without coming to the end of that from which we would subtract.

Thus we see that uranium, or thorium, after having discharged its rays for a long period, is so changed that we recognize it as radium. Radium, in turn, after exhausting a certain degree of its radioactive powers, becomes lead. For instance, we know that uranium, being the heaviest element, would be number 92 in the scale of atomic numbers, with an atomic weight of 238·14. Thorium, number 90, has an atomic weight of 232·12 and is so similar in some phases of its nature to uranium that it is also a source of radium ; it stands in the atomic scale as 88 with an atomic weight of 225·97. Lead has an atomic number of 82 with an atomic weight of 207·22. The differing atomic weights of these substances demonstrate Einstein's statement regarding the change of mass equalling the change in energy.

We have spoken before of *homœopathy in its relation to fundamental laws*, and this chapter is an attempt to set forth further deductions on that basis.

Thus we comprehend that every step toward understanding of the working of the natural laws brings us to a clearer vision of a few basic cosmic laws, fundamentally few in number but with a multiplicity of manifestations. The laws governing homœopathy are seemingly not closely associated with laws governing other forms of "pure science", yet the knowledge is borne in upon us that this is one manifestation of that which is basic ; it differs only in its manifestation and not in its essence. We must teach

ourselves to discriminate between the multiple manifestations (or applications of the law) through differing forms—as
they appear to casual observation—and their essences, which
are so closely similar as to lead us to question if they be not
fundamentally identical.

Sir J. C. Bose, from whose invaluable records we have
quoted from time to time, quotes from ancient Hindu
philosophy a throbbing, vital truth to which every thoughtful
homœopathic physician can subscribe and that he must
heed :

THEY WHO SEE BUT ONE, IN ALL THE CHANGING MANIFOLD-
NESS OF THIS UNIVERSE, UNTO THEM BELONGS ETERNAL
TRUTH—UNTO NONE ELSE, UNTO NONE ELSE.

CHAPTER VIII

TAKING THE CASE

(SEE *Organon*, Paragraphs 83-104.) In taking the case, the homœopathic physician has two objects in view. First, there is the object of diagnosis. This is to place your difficulty in a group class. The homœopathic physician can have no other object in making a diagnosis than to classify the symptoms under a group head, since the homœopathic physician never uses his diagnosis for therapeutic purposes. In this he differs from the ordinary school of medicine, which uses the diagnosis as a guide to the desired therapy, certain group conditions determined by the diagnosis determining the therapy to be applied.

With the homœopathic physician, the group is never treated as a unit ; the individual patient, into whatever diagnostic group he may fall, is treated as an individual, and the therapeutic measures are directed according to the individual symptoms.

Therefore, the second and greater object in taking the case is to select the true symptoms of the patient, and to clarify them so that we can make a definite picture of the ills of the patient.

Many of the things of which we speak, when it comes to taking the case, may seem very commonplace, but there is nothing in the practice of homœopathy upon which so much depends as the thorough comprehension of the background that we must have in taking the case, and getting the case properly before us for analysis. The presentation of the case should include the whole picture. We cannot depend upon our memory in taking the case. The picture must be preserved in indelible form, in a form which we may go over in review without the danger of leaving out any important symptom ; we must be able to turn back to any individual symptom or group of symptoms at any time. So as the first requisite in taking the case, you must have your record cards with you to note down the case as it is taken. So much depends upon this record that you cannot afford not to take the time for properly recording the case.

In making the first prescription, this record is all-important ; and in the making of subsequent prescriptions and in reviewing the case so that we may know the sequence of symptoms and the order of disappearance of the symptoms, we cannot move with any degree of assurance unless we have the record in accessible form.

The attitude of the physician should be one of absolute rest and poise, with no preconceived ideas nor prejudices. He should be in a quiet, listening attitude, and as the case is presented to him he should have no previous impressions as to what remedy the patient will require, because this of itself would bias his judgment.

The first thing to note is the patient's name, age, sex, vocation and, if possible, avocation. Then we are often greatly helped by getting a record of the family ; that is, the age of the parents, their general health, and cause of death if they are deceased. This applies to brothers and sisters also ; and we must not neglect to get a picture of the types of ailments from which they have suffered. We often get a good picture of hereditary tendencies in this way. Find out, if possible, if there is or has been blood relationships between ancestors. Consanguinity plays an important part in hereditary tendencies as well as in making your prescription (Phos.).

Now we are ready to proceed with the record of the patient himself. Let us begin to record his past illnesses. What illnesses has he had ? How about his recovery from each illness ? Particularly note whether he reports himself as fully recovering from illnesses, or whether he says he " has not been well since " any particular illness.

Now ask the patient to tell you in his own words how he became ill and exactly how he feels. Do not offer any interruption, lest you break his thread of thought. As you record the symptoms, leave space between them so that you can fill in later answers to questions as it may be necessary. If he comes to a point where he seems to hesitate, simply ask, " What else ? " Continue this system of interested listening until he (seemingly) has exhausted his story.

Then you are ready to review the case as it has been given to you. Perhaps before we go into the next step, the questioning by the doctor, it will be well to state the things we must NEVER do. We cannot place too much emphasis upon the absolute necessity of leaving these things undone.

1. Avoid all leading questions. By leading questions, I mean questions that suggest answers to the patient, or suggest that you want to bring out certain answers. Some patients are desperately anxious to have answers suggested to them and the physician must be constantly on his guard to avoid doing so.

2. Never ask direct questions, that may be answered with a direct affirmative or negative.

3. Never ask alternating questions.

4. Avoid questioning along the line of a remedy. Sometimes we may get a clue from the statement of a symptom that may suggest a certain remedy, and we must be very cautious not to allow this to prejudice us in favour of the remedy suggested by questioning the patient along this line, and thus perhaps bias the patient in his replies.

5. While you are dealing with one symptom, confine yourself to that symptom. Never skip from one symptom to another at random, as it confuses the patient and scatters the physician's ideas.

Now we will return to the necessity of rounding out the symptom picture in our record. Some symptoms may have been given with a fair degree of completeness ; others are very incomplete. We must complete, as far as possible, every symptom that has been presented, and for this careful questioning is necessary. Each symptom must be rounded out as to time and place ; the sensations ; the kind of distress ; the type of pain ; all of the modalities connected with it ; the probable causation, that is, what the patient thinks was the start of the trouble. Under the modalities, we must secure the aggravations and ameliorations of each individual symptom, so far as possible. Not the least important is the emotional reaction of the patient.

When we work out the recording of the case in this way,

we cover all the parts of the man, and can see the picture as a whole. We must leave nothing uncovered. In order to do this, we may have to bring into play the testimony of the family or nurse on symptoms or conditions that may have a bearing of considerable value. However, this source of information must always be scanned with a great deal of circumspection and we must weigh the integrity of the source as being worthy of consideration.

With the most careful recording and the most cautious questioning we may be unable to find complete symptoms and may be unable to build up more than a sketch of the patient himself. We will deal with this in a later chapter.

In acute illnesses, take the acute symptoms, carefully record each one, and find out all there is to know about them. Likewise in the chronic picture, record all the symptoms as far back as you can dig out the symptoms, and the sequence of the symptom pictures, and prescribe for that state. However, if you are dealing with an acute condition, limit yourself to dealing with the acute state alone and do not at the same time attempt to dip into what has been a chronic state. Acute manifestations show themselves with surprising clearness, and to include chronic symptoms that have been manifest at other periods will but confuse the picture.

Remember, we must prescribe for the totality of the symptom picture and not for any one symptom alone, but for the complete picture as it is presented in the individual. In an acute explosion the chronic picture will retreat completely ; therefore, in treating the complete picture that is present there will be no need to take the chronic picture into consideration. At the close of the acute attack we again see the chronic picture. Then will be the time to deal with it. In fact, there is no time in the history of the case when we can see the picture of the chronic underlying condition so plainly as at the end of an acute attack, after the acute conditions have subsided. Therefore, after dealing properly with the acute attack, and waiting until it subsides, we will be in a position to see clearly the picture of the chronic case. This condition following acute illness is much more apt to be the manifestation of the chronic condition than it is to be the aftermath of acute conditions, as is popularly supposed.

In considering the totality we cannot over-emphasize the necessity of getting the complete description of each symptom, as to its location, character, and modalities. The modalities, the aggravations and ameliorations, are the most important. Next in order come the character of the sensations.

The most important symptoms, of course, are the general symptoms that pertain to the patient as a whole. Then come the aggravations and ameliorations. The mental symptoms rank very highly for the reason that they point to the man himself, and they may be classed under the generals to a marked degree.

The thorough examination of the patient from every possible angle should be carried through, not for the gross diagnostic symptoms, important as these may be from diagnostic and hygienic points of view. From the curative point of view we should not fail to elicit all the possible clues that may lead us to the remedy. Subjective and objective symptoms are to be elicited and recorded. Sometimes this will require the utmost ingenuity to elicit the necessary intelligent replies without leading questions. The physician's degree of success in obtaining the proper symptom picture lies in his skill and patience. We cannot rush these patients through. We must be good listeners. Get the patient to talking, and tactfully keep him talking about the symptoms rather than wandering far afield. Then cultivate your powers of listening and give your powers of observation full sway, to form the complete picture of the little details and habits of your patient. It has been said that criminal lawyers should be medical men ; it is eminently necessary, however, that homœopathic physicians be past masters of the art of cross-examination ; and the observance of the patient's every movement and expression should be a matter of record.

Before leaving the case, go over again the family history, the personal history, the mental and physical symptoms. Consider the temperament, the habits, the occupation, the personality of the patient. Ask yourself if you have skipped anything. See that you have questioned every item, every function ; question the modalities in particular. Go over the previous drug treatment and consider that. Remember that the nature and sensations of the symptoms, the time of day, the positions and circumstances under which symptoms appear, are the most important modifiers of any given case.

To clarify these general instructions, let us take up the matter in greater detail, and go over together the following requirements :

In chronic work it is necessary to take into consideration the general symptoms. By general symptoms we mean those symptoms which pertain to the patient as a whole, or to the complaint which he brings to us. In order to get a complete picture of the case as a whole let us consider these elements:

The aggravations, the periodicity, the seasonal aggravations, weather aggravations as to sun, wind, cold, dry, wet, fog, etc. ; changes of weather, as cold to warm or warm to cold ; changes of weather as before, during or after storms, such as thunderstorms, rain, snow, etc. ; the tendency to develop certain conditions, such as the tendency to take cold, sore throats, headaches, etc. ; the reactions to fresh air, such as craving for or aggravation from ; reactions to positions in rest or in action, such as < walking, or > lying with arms raised ; these reactions in relation to position include also riding in trains, in cars, in vessels ; conditions of appetite and the cravings or aversions of aggravations from certain foods ; the effects of vaccination or serum treatment ; reactions to bathing ; effect of altitude, seashore, or mountain ; the amount of clothing required, during the day and at night ; the rapidity with which wounds heal ; if the patient is subject to hæmorrhages ; the reaction of the patient to the presence of others, whether he prefers to be alone or in company, or whether < being alone or in assembly; the sides affected.

How about the thermic reactions of the patient ? Is he hot or cold, in general or under varying circumstances ? If there are variations of temperature do they involve the whole or a part of the body ? Is his skin moist or dry ? If he perspires, under what conditions ? Freely or scantily All over or only in certain parts ? Is the perspiration offensive, exhausting, greasy, hot or cold ? Is he better or worse during or after ? How is the sweat related in time to the chill and heat ? Is the chill (or heat) partial or general ? Is there shivering of a part or in general, and does this occur with or without chill ? Is there thirst ? In what relation of time to the heat, chill and or sweat ?

Note should be made of the aversions and cravings ; the type of sleep and dreams ; the positions of the body in sleep ; how the patient wakens from sleep and his condition after waking. With either a man or woman patient, the abnormalities of the sexual functions should be noted. Then the strange, rare, and peculiar symptoms should be sought out.

I have left until the last mention of the essential part of the case-taking, the comprehension of the mental symptoms. To a great extent these are symptoms that must be observed from the attitude of the patient. Another reason for leaving these until the last is that during the examination you have probably been able to get the confidence of your patients to a greater degree and they will give you more fully their confidence. Find if they are subject to hallucinations or fixed ideas, especially any fears that are persistent. Take into consideration irritability, or a change in disposition ; if you can unearth traits of jealousy, or absent-mindedness, these must be seriously considered. Sadness, ailments arising from grief, vexation, sudden joy, are important. Is the patient over-insistent upon the minor details of life as to scrupulous cleanliness, etc. ? Or is the contrary true ?

Your patient should readily reveal many of these most important things to you if you have been tactful and have secured his confidence.

I refer you to a wonderful questionnaire compiled by Dr. Pierre Schmidt. This will assist you in securing the information you desire, and if you will study this carefully it will prove a valuable guide in directing your questioning, *after the patient has finished telling you all he thought was necessary to your treatment of the case.*

It is well to reiterate the instruction : Do not interrupt your patient while he is telling all he knows of his case, except in so far as he may require guidance to keep him to the subject in hand. The physician's questioning comes afterward, and it is here that we must complete the picture of the case.

What are the essentials to record in taking the case ? (*Answer :* The general symptoms ; the modalities ; the sensations ; the concomitants.)

Why should we have a written record of each case ? (*Answer :* So that we may view the case as a complete whole, (1) for our first prescription ; (2) for future reference, so that we may note progress.)

Why do we need to pay little attention to the chronic symptoms in taking an acute case ? (*Answer :* We take each case as completely as possible, for when an acute seizure is present the chronic symptoms usually retire into the background, so that we need only prescribe for the totality as presented.)

When do we find the chronic symptoms portrayed most clearly ? (*Answer :* At the end of an acute attack the chronic symptoms usually show themselves clearly, even more clearly than at other times ; the conditions following an acute attack are not the result of the acute attack, but because Nature has cleared the patient to a greater or less degree by the acute explosion and this leaves a clear picture of the chronic condition.)

CHAPTER IX

ANALYSIS OF THE CASE

IN analysis of the case, the value of symptoms must be taken into consideration on several points. First, the personality, the individuality of the patient, must stand out pre-eminently in the picture. This can be illustrated by likening the whole symptomatology to a complete picture of the whole individual, a whole personality. This embraces not only his physical characteristics, but the expression of his mental and emotional characteristics as well.

While the generals rank the highest in evaluating the case, and without generals we cannot expect to find the *simillimum*, the mental and emotional characteristics have a high value, since these are the true reflections of his personality, the man himself. Because the subjective symptoms are the registration of his physical or other difficulties as expressed upon his own personality, these are also of great value. The objective symptoms are less differentiative, yet their value lies in the fact that they cannot be distorted by the design of the patient ; he little realizes that he is manifesting these objective symptoms and therefore they picture accurately certain phases of the case.

Objective symptoms, those that are seen by the careful observer, have more importance in child life than in adult life, because through them we see the expression of the child's disposition and desires. Therefore, many of the seemingly objective symptoms may be translated into subjective form. It is for us to interpret the symptom according to our understanding of its proper value. While they may be presented to us in child life almost entirely as objective symptoms, yet they may have their counterpart subjectively in the provings.

Now in taking a case we must take into consideration the nature of the disease and its peculiar types. We must know disease accurately before we can give effective relief.

Occasional cures take place without such knowledge, but it is almost by accident. That is, we must know its peculiar manifestations in each individual case, taking into consideration its complete symptom totality. The complete knowledge of the case is associated with another important item. We must know and possess the means by which we are able to relieve. Without this latter knowledge any knowledge of symptoms is of no avail.

There has been a great knowledge of disease attained from investigators from the earliest times ; methods have been improved whereby diagnostic symptoms have been correlated, and all praise is due to these investigators along this line. The only difficulty is that diseases have come to be treated by names of the diseases instead of by individual symptoms ; the disease has been treated rather than the patient. It is only upon the totality of the symptoms that we can base our prescription, and so we require many individual symptoms as showing the characteristics and personality of the patient ; so these diagnostic symptoms are of very little use to the homœopathic prescriber in selecting the remedy. In fact, the *simillimum* is practically never found among the diagnostic symptoms. In considering the diagnostic symptoms in the selection of the remedy, its only practical value is in excluding those remedies from consideration which do not correspond to the genius of the disease, but act chiefly on other parts of the organism.

If we allow ourselves to become influenced by the diagnosis in making our remedy selection, we are very apt to become confused and fail to help our patient. We may be faced with a diagnosis of some grave condition such as some form of deep abscess, a grave pneumonia condition, an internal hæmorrhage, or any one of a host of conditions. Selection of the remedy on the basis of the diagnosis may, and probably will, fail completely. However, the symptoms of the patient are an infallible guide, and the more serious the condition, the clearer cut are the indications for the remedy. If we allow ourselves to be guided by these symptoms, we shall probably save the patient, *even though the remedy selected on the basis of the symptom totality may never have been used under like diagnostic conditions before.*

The symptoms of location frequently furnish quite characteristic symptoms, and they deserve particular attention, since every remedy acts more, and more decidedly, on certain parts of the organism. These differences enter into the consideration of certain local manifestations, like furunculosis, but it also enters into those types of diseases that localize in certain parts, like gout in the great toe, and yet are of systemic origin. These symptoms all have their bearing and should be considered as to location ; and they are particularly valuable to us as pertaining to localization in the right or left side of the body, or of certain organs of the body. They are particularly valuable in noticing the location, as in the base or apices or middle lobe of the lungs. They are particularly to be noticed as to direction ; on which side the trouble starts and in which direction the symptoms move and where they localize, as, for instance, throat troubles going from the left side to the right, or the right side to the left, or continuous alternation of sides.

All these finer shadings have much to do with homœopathy, and have very little to do with ordinary medicine. Even the nurses wonder when we ask regarding the localization of symptoms. However, these things do enter in and make considerable difference in our ability to select the correct homœopathic remedy. The localization of symptoms and the direction of symptoms will often appear as marked symptoms before pathological changes have manifested themselves, as for instance, in the beginning of the syndrome which we call tonsillitis, or in the beginning of a similar syndrome in pneumonic conditions where, if the remedy is given an early opportunity to exhibit its power, the pathological condition will not arise. In such states the localization and direction of symptoms become of considerable moment to the homœopathic physician.

The chief aim of the homœopathic physician consists in ascertaining the remedy that most completely and fully covers each individual case. In other words, the totality of the symptoms. We hear so much of the totality of the symptoms that sometimes it behoves us to stop and think what this means. The homœopathic physician may be likened to an artist painting a portrait. He fills in all those features pertaining to the likeness which he is painting, and those features which may be found on all faces, eyes, ears, nose, mouth, lips. In this way all individuals are similar, but each individual has peculiarities of his own, and in order to make the picture complete the artist must present the individualities in the portrait, but not accentuate over and above the other features the normal position, shape, and size as it appears in the individual himself. In taking a likeness, how strange the finished picture would be were we to draw or paint only the peculiar things ! Just a nose or just an eye, and nothing by which we could distinguish the one whom the picture was intended to represent. On the other hand, if we painted the classic features only there would be no distinguishing characteristics in the finished product.

It is in this relationship that we must gain a knowledge of the concomitant symptoms if we would prescribe homœopathically. In drawing the picture we must present the rare, the striking, the peculiar symptoms which present themselves, not out of keeping but associated with the other symptoms which form a background upon which the peculiar, rare, and characteristic symptoms must be presented as determining the individuality, the personality, of the man for whom we are prescribing. It is not the common symptoms, common to all disease syndromes, that are of value, but the rare, the peculiar, the unusual, that stand out by themselves. It must necessarily follow that these concomitant symptoms have a wide variety and are widely distributed throughout the organism.

It is almost impossible to name all the peculiarities in all the cases that we might find, but there are certain ones that stand out. First of all, those symptoms that are common and found in almost all diseases may be left out of our count unless they manifest themselves in a striking manner. The same may be true of those ailments and symptoms that usually appear in the disease under consideration, unless they should be distinguished by some rare peculiarity, and in this way offer something particularly characteristic, like thirstless fever, or chill with desire to uncover. On the other hand, all the attendant symptoms should be carefully noted :

(a) Those symptoms which rarely appear in connection

with the leading disease, and therefore are found rarely among the provings.

(b) Those which belong to another sphere of disease than the principal ailment.

(c) Those which have more or less characteristic signs of the medicine even though they have not before been noticed in the present relationship or diagnostic group.

Then again, besides these concomitant symptoms that have already been mentioned, there should be one in which the genius of the remedy should be plainly and definitely portrayed, so that it would be immediately noticeable. This symptom would immediately attain such importance that it would outweigh the chief ailment, and thus be chosen as the *simillimum*. Such a *simillimum* corresponds to Hahnemann's dictum which calls for a striking, strange, peculiar, and unusual sign, which may then be considered almost alone in choosing the remedy, because it gives pre-eminently the character of the whole design.

A peculiar and unusual deduction from these concomitant symptoms is that they often illumine remedies that have never been thought of before in this relationship to the individual case and therefore broaden our vision and concept of the LAW OF SIMILARS.

In considering what Hahnemann calls the " strange, rare, and peculiar (characteristic) symptoms " and their value in directing us to the remedy, let us remember the exposition that A. Conan Doyle so often puts into the mouth of his famous character, Sherlock Holmes. This worthy, in summing up some famous case in which he has acted the scientific detective, uses these words : " That which is out of the common is usually a guide rather than a hindrance." And again : " That which seemingly confuses the case is the very thing that furnishes the clue to its solution."

In considering the value of symptoms in solving any chronic case we cannot do better than to take these aphorisms for our guide, and to remember that those symptoms which confuse the ordinary physician, or which he regards as useless or as having no relationship to the case, are the very symptoms that furnish the clues for the remedy.

In considering the value of symptoms there are certain

symptoms that are apparently caused by conditions, and that almost precede the symptomatology, and seem to give a basis for the patient's condition. These may be exposure to cold ; exposure to wet ; all those conditions of which people say that thus and so was the cause of their illness and the cause of their symptoms. These play a large part in pathological prescribing. In pathological prescribing these causes of disease loom large ; in homœopathic prescribing they do not loom as large, save as showing the tendencies of the patient.

This embraces causes that are directly traceable to diet as well as climatic conditions. Embraced in this category also are susceptibility to disease conditions and idiosyncrasies. The symptoms that are produced by trade conditions come in this category and the poisonings that may take place from too much drugging, or from working in metals. The symptoms produced from such conditions may be valuable in showing the pathological trend of the metal or gas or drug causing the condition, but they do not show the finer differentiations nor have they the same value that they do from the exhibition of the potencies.

Sometimes these early symptoms will place the physician in a position to see clearly the basic miasmatic condition from which the patient is himself suffering. This should bear a large place in the evaluation of symptoms.

This, too, brings up the question of infectious diseases and the symptomatology attending the so-called contagious diseases. It is the duty of the physician to take very close observation of the first cases he has in an epidemic of infectious diseases, for the symptomatology of each epidemic is distinct of the epidemic, while the next epidemic may have an entirely different symptomatology. Immunity can be assured to patients if we will closely observe the symptomatology and select the epidemic remedy in the early stages of each epidemic, by administering the epidemic remedy as a prophylactic. In this way the symptomatology of epidemic diseases is exceedingly valuable to the homœopathic physician.

In analysing the case, very valuable symptoms are those pertaining to the aggravations and ameliorations, because the aggravations and ameliorations are the natural modifiers of diseased states and are the definite reaction of the man himself. We must take into consideration that every symptom of note has these modifying conditions of aggravation and amelioration, as to time, the time of day, the time of season, the time of the moon ; the aggravation or amelioration from thermic conditions ; from motion or rest, of the part affected or of the condition as a whole ; from lying down or sitting or standing, and the positions taken during such conditions, waking or sleeping, and the aggravation and amelioration from such positions and circumstances ; the various positions in motion that aggravate or ameliorate ; the desires or aversions to eating and drinking, especially in feverish conditions ; aggravations from certain foods and drink. These are all modifications that are of the utmost importance in evaluating the symptoms.

While we cannot hope to cure a patient without strong general symptoms, yet conditions of aggravation or amelioration may in themselves become generals, if they appertain in the same way to several parts of the body ; they then become conditions of the man as a whole, or general symptoms, even though they seemingly express themselves in local parts. For instance, if a headache is < by motion ; if the pain in the knee is < by walking or stepping ; if there is pain in the shoulder from raising the arm ; then the < from motion becomes a general as of the whole man, although it seemingly appears in dissociated parts.

The contradictory symptoms have an importance, because they may rule out many of the remedies that otherwise might be considered in connection with an individual case. That is, symptoms that are decidedly opposed to the provings, like the thirstlessness of the fever of *Ignatia* or *Apis* or *Pulsatilla* when fever is present and when other symptoms agree. Contradictory symptoms may have a strong bearing in choosing the remedy from the standpoint of being themselves a symptom, just as a paucity of symptoms may be a symptom in itself, as has been brought out in the provings of the so-called " do nothing " remedies, which are often called for in profound states. For this reason, if you cannot find a remedy because of alternating or contradictory symptoms, or for very lack of symptoms, take these conditions as indications for symptoms of the very first rank.

To emphasize again the necessity for consideration of the aggravations and ameliorations of the periods of distress : it is well to bear in mind the period of onset in periodic manifestations of symptoms, the increase, the acme, the decrease, and the end of disease manifestations in the evaluation of symptoms. For instance, conditions such as *Cedron, Spigelia, Sanguinaria, Natrum mur.*—these remedies have a decided periodicity, and it is very important to consider also those symptoms that occur in the recession or in the intervals between the periods of aggravation.

These are but a few of the conditions confronting the homœopathic physician if he would cure his patients, and he should learn early to evaluate symptoms, because symptoms are the sole expression of the internal disturbance, and it is only by the proper understanding of these expressions in disease, and an equal knowledge of the condition as expressed in the provings, that we can apply our guiding law, *similia similibus curentur*, intelligently and for the benefit of our patients.

What symptoms rank the highest in an analysis of the case ?

How do we rate : Generals ? Mental and emotional symptoms ? Subjective symptoms ? Objective symptoms ? Concomitant symptoms ?

Where do we place much emphasis on objective symptoms and why ?

Cite an instance where an objective symptom may be translated as a subjective symptom.

How much consideration should we place on the diagnosis of the case ?

Give an outline of the totality of a case.

When may common symptoms attain a peculiar value ?

What do we mean by " epidemic remedy " and how can we determine the epidemic remedy ?

When may a particular symptom become a general ?

CHAPTER X

THE LAW OF CURE

ALL natural forces are based upon law. These laws do not operate in a limited field, but are universal. To illustrate, the law of gravitation is not limited in its scope to the earth, but its influence extends throughout the universe.

Hahnemann, by his fine observation and the inductive method of reasoning, became convinced of the law of cure, *similia similibus curentur*, and embraced it and declared it to be universal, a basic law of therapeutics.

If there is any general law of cure, that law must express some relationship between the medicine and the disease. To be of any practical use such a relationship must be exhibited, and we must be able to demonstrate such a relation between a disease and its remedy that any examination of the former shall determine the latter. Nothing can be known of the disease save through the phenomena known as symptoms ; these are evident to our observation and senses and must be recognized. These phenomena represent the individuality of the disease in the only way in which we can recognize it. A corresponding capability exists in the drug, of producing an individual, although artificial, disease, which we recognize through the same method of observing the phenomena produced after the administration of the drug. The power to produce these phenomena is what we call the properties of the drug.

It is the characteristic of disease to produce certain phenomena which are not observable in perfect health. This is true whether the changes are functional or structural ; what we recognize as symptoms are all that can be known of the disease. It is only through the observation of these expressions that we can make any use of the law of cure, and there can be no general consideration of the rule of cure unless it comprises a consideration of symptoms as one of the necessary elements. One might say that a comprehension of the symptoms of a given case was one of the primary factors, and in so far as one comprehends the expression of disease in these phenomena is one equipped to follow the law of cure in any particular case. Symptoms are the only representative expression of the diseased state. We include sensations as expressed by the patient, the appearances in all parts of the body, the varied circumstances under which these symptoms were recorded, and the varied grouping of these symptoms, in any consideration of the case.

When a symptom is noted under certain circumstances and not under others, this obvious relation between the symptom and its related circumstance is in itself a symptom, or rather, a part of the symptom, the sensation being quite incomplete without the expressed relationship of circumstance. Very often the concomitant of circumstance is of greater importance to the whole case than the expressed sensation, but the sensation is much more frequently expressed by the patient.

Two or more symptoms may appear together, or synchronize with each other, so frequently that they are really one symptom and must be considered as such in our analysis. As nothing in nature can be represented by a single property, so no disease can be represented by a single symptom.

A law of cure must represent some relation between the properties of a disease and the medicinal qualities of a drug ; or in other words, we must have some concept of the character of the drug's action on the living body that will interpret the law of cure in the action of disease.

This character of the drug is represented, not by a single effect, but by a group of effects. This group of effects is the only representation we have or can have of the medicinal character of a drug on the living body, and since these same effects are found in disease states, these effects are the only relationship that can be established between the medicinal effects of a drug and disease. *There can be no law of cure unless it expresses some definite relation between these two groups, or classes.*

The homœopathic law establishes a definite relation, not only between proved drugs and known diseases, but between all the unexplored medical wealth and the undeveloped requirements of sickness. Like the law of gravitation, the law of cure as taught by Hahnemann is not, and cannot be, limited to a small group of conditions ; the limitations rest entirely with our ignorance. Hahnemann and his followers constitute the only group of medical philosophers who have always been true to the inductive method of reasoning, and by scientifically following this method of reasoning, based upon known facts, they have established this law of therapeutics.

It has been proven by experience that a medicine will remove a group of symptoms similar to the group which it is capable of producing. This law, founded upon observation of facts, has been the product of inductive reasoning and has been proven by years of experience to be true and sure.

No medicine can cure any disease unless it acts upon all the diseased parts, either directly or indirectly. The more similar the symptoms of a drug resemblance to the disease, the nearer is its vital approach to the disease, and the more dynamic its action. The number of parts of the human body susceptible of receiving the curative action of drugs vastly outnumbers those recognized in the anatomy, because disease and cure do not lie in the tisues except as a reflection of the man himself. This we may see from the almost infinite diversity of symptoms producible and curable by drugs. There is an almost infinite number of parts or cells in each organ, and this vast number are suffering together, some more or some less ; the affection of each element may be different from that of any other, the aggregate affection composing the disease of that tissue of that one organ. How much more complicated is the disease of the whole body, even though that manifestation be classed as a " local disease " ! One organ cannot suffer alone any more than one cell can suffer by itself. Every disease affects in some way and to some degree every organ, every tissue, every molecule.

Because of custom we express ourselves in this sense as from the greater toward the smaller, from without inward, yet an analytical study must remind us that the disease manifestation is an exfoliation, an outward manifestation of an inward turmoil, that is not found in the most minute examination known to man of any cell or portion of the human frame. We may find disease manifestations, but we cannot find disease itself.

No medicine can effect a perfect cure unless it has a curative action upon every diseased part, and in just the proportion that each part manifests disorder. Potentized medicine, administered according to the law of *similia*, is the true regulator of the vital energy, that vital essence which is synonymous, or at least analogous, to the man himself and lies very close to life itself.

The totality of any disease is the totality of the morbid action, sensations and manifestations ; any true and complete and comprehensive law of therapeutics must recognize all the morbid phenomena and show some relation between them and the curative agent. This relationship must be direct and clear.

Joslin says the degrees of conceivable relationship between the action of drugs and that of disease may be represented by an immense circle. Identity is the central point, and on this point stands *isopathy*. Immediately around it are arranged the most perfect degrees of similarity. This is the province of *homœopathy*, the *simillimum*. Contiguous to this is the ring of similarities, less perfect but still great ; this field is the field of the near similar but not the *simillimum*.

Isopathy is not homœopathy ; we must keep this distinction ever before us. Isopathy is identity ; homœopathy rests its whole case on the similarity, and in the degree of its perfection we may be sure of the results.

We cannot be accused of combating symptoms ; rather, we are guided by symptoms in combating disease.

The law of cure, *similia similibus curentur*, is as fundamental as any law in nature. It is a law of universal adaptability to human sickness ; it ranks in the field of medicine with Newton's law of gravitation in the field of astronomy. This is the only general law for the cure of the physical and mental ills of man ; it is the only method of healing that depends, as a whole, upon one general principle, and it is the only method of healing that has continued to withstand the pressure of time and changing circumstances. It is a law of nature, discovered by following the thread of inductive reasoning, and proven to be true by countless tests.

What is the most we can hope to know of disease ?

What can we know of drug action ?

What part does observation play in homœopathic prescribing ?

What kind of symptoms are most frequently voiced by the patient ? (*Answer* : Sensations.)

What are concomitant symptoms, and how do you rank them as to relative value ?

Why do we say : The homœopathic law establishes a definite relation between drugs and disease ?

What are disease manifestations ?

What is the difference between isopathy and homœopathy ?

Chapter XI

THE CHIEF COMPLAINT AND THE AUXILIARY SYMPTOMS IN THEIR RELATION TO THE CASE

ALMOST every case that comes to the attention of the physician presents two distinct phases, two separate parts, as it were : the part comprising the symptoms of which the patient complains, those which are most annoying to him and most outstanding in his recognition ; and secondly, those symptoms which he does not recognize as symptoms or which he does not consider worth reporting or does not consider as having any relationship to the case.

The chief complaint has a psychological value out of all proportion to its value in homœopathic prescribing : it brings the patient to the physician, and if the physician responds and by careful questioning draws out the history of other symptoms, the patient feels a satisfaction and confidence that the physician is not treating his case as of no consequence.

Now the chief complaint is a very necessary part of every case ; some of our colleges are giving the chief complaint of every case much consideration. The young physician places much dependence upon this part of the case ; it is close to his training along diagnostic lines. The older prescriber, while giving due weight to the chief symptoms, feels that in prescribing he must consider the totality of the symptoms and in order to do so he must give more weight to the other part, probably unexpressed without some encouragement on the part of the physician, which is an even more necessary part of the case than the chief complaint, because it is that part which manifests more clearly the individuality of the patient and indicates most clearly the individuality of the remedy to cover the case—the totality of the symptoms, if you prefer.

The chief complaint, as presented by the patient, may be altogether different in value from the symptoms discovered and illuminated by the physician's analysis of the case. The chief complaint is often a pathological state, or an approach toward a pathological state, in the functional sphere.

The chief complaint, or the leading symptoms, may be defined as those symptoms for which there is clear pathological foundation ; or the symptoms that are most prominent and clearly recognizable ; or the symptoms which first attract the attention of the patient or physician ; or which cause the most suffering ; or which indicate definitely the seat and nature of the morbid process ; which form the " warp of the fabric ", as it has been expressed.

The auxiliary or concomitant symptom or group of symptoms seldom has any definite relationship to the leading symptoms from the standpoint of theoretical pathology ; these are the symptoms which the pathologist would exclude as accidental and meaningless, but they have actually a definite relationship to the case, because they occur in the same patient, and at the same time or in definite relationship of time, as the other symptoms which are considered the chief complaint. If they do not fit into the theories of pathology, they have an even greater individual value in the case ; those symptoms which can be explained are of little help in selecting the homœopathic remedy, but it is this group of auxiliary or concomitant symptoms which limit the choice of the *simillimum*.

That group of which the patient complains most, almost without exception cannot be relied upon for the definite selection of the remedy ; it is the concomitant group of symptoms which, taken in conjunction with the major group of symptoms, makes possible the definite selection of the remedy by greatly reducing the number of remedies indicated in such conditions, and upon a closer analysis we can pick the *simillimum* unerringly from this small group.

For instance, when we find a case where the patient gives as her chief complaint ovarian pain, we cannot instantly pick the remedy from a consideration of this symptom alone ; the homœopathic materia medica has over fifty remedies that have this symptom. Cerebral congestion may be met with any one of 150 or more remedies ; and so with many single symptom pictures. We might cite numerous complaints where the chief complaint would lead us into a morass of remedies, any one of which *might* give relief to the patient, but only one of which would cure.

At times the chief complaint seems contradictory to the auxiliary group of symptoms brought out by the physician's questioning ; the patient may have, within the course of a day, an exceedingly dry mouth, and then complain of its excessive moisture. The patient may complain of diarrhœa, but a careful taking of the case may reveal an alternation of diarrhœa and constipation. Or there may be a complete alteration of symptoms at different seasons of the year, as rheumatic conditions at one time, and gastric disturbances at another time ; rheumatic pains in the limbs during one attack, and perhaps rheumatic iritis at another time. The physician will find many such alternating symptom groups, any one of which may be the chief complaint. Only the thoughtless physician will tell the patient that the present symptom group is the one to be considered at the present time, and when the other symptom group appears it will be plenty of time to consider that group. Such an attitude on the part of the physician may seem logical, but the thoughtful student of homœopathy realizes that many remedies in our materia medica have alternating group symptoms, and he cannot ignore any symptoms which the patient may recite.

Much has been said of keynote prescribing ; many at the present time use a repertory simply as a means of seeking a key to unlock the case through the peculiar and unusual symptom. This has a certain value, if we are so fortunate as to find the *simillimum* by some outstandingly peculiar symptom ; but most often this is not enough, and it has little more value than selecting at random any one remedy from a group known to have a certain symptom in the provings. *We must not fail to recognize the value of the totality of the symptoms* ; and this must take into consideration the chief complaints, those of which the patient most often complains, plus the peculiar characteristics of the patient. If both these elements are present, we may be sure we are on the right track.

Let us consider a few cases.

A young woman complains of tension, stiffness and lameness through the muscles of her back, particularly between the shoulders and in the nape of the neck, the stiffness causing a pulling sensation of the muscles even into the cheeks. She cannot turn her head without distress ; bending the body or raising the arms, especially the left, aggravates the condition. How many remedies and what remedies flash through your mind as possibly covering these symptoms ? However, you feel the need of more careful questioning to elicit more characteristic symptoms, for this symptom group, although it is the chief complaint is not enough on which to base your prescription if you wish to be sure of curing your patient.

It develops upon further inquiry that she also has a leucorrhoea. This symptom also might come into a number of remedies that you have already hastily considered as applicable to the case, but in itself it has no value as a differentiating symptom. Upon careful questioning, the patient volunteered that her leucorrhoea comes on only when sitting ; she is absolutely free from it as soon as she gets up on her feet, either standing or walking. Here is a truly auxiliary symptom that has a unique value : *Leucorrhoea only when sitting*.

So far as I have been able to determine, there is only one remedy which in the provings has developed this characteristic symptom, and that is *Fagopyrum*. Lest we be accused of keynote prescribing, let us look over the symptoms of this remedy in their relationship to the chief complaint.

We find the muscular tension and drawing, especially between the shoulders and in the nape. We find other symptoms of which the patient complained, less characteristic of any remedy in particular than those mentioned, and then we find the outstanding symptom, characteristic and peculiar, which is perhaps the most characteristic and peculiar symptom of *Fagopyrum*, the leucorrhoea only while sitting ; and we know beyond any question that we have found the *simillimum*.

In this case the chief complaint was the tension of the muscles, the lameness ; but the outstanding concomitant symptom that apparently bore no relationship to the chief complaint was the leucorrhoea > while standing or walking, < sitting. It was the concomitant symptom which, taken in conjunction with the other more common symptoms, defined the choice of the remedy.

A case of chronic asthma complains of the characteristic wheezing, suffocative sensation and other symptoms which we call asthma. How can we prescribe on these symptoms? How many remedies have these symptoms? Of course, the answer is that the chief complaint here is of use merely as a background upon which to depict the individual peculiarities in the case. His cough is < at night; he is > after expectoration; his hands and feet are icy cold. These symptoms may limit the number of remedies that we consider, but still there is nothing that definitely points the way to the selection of the remedy. He adds that he has an attack come on after he becomes angry, or the attack is < after anger; < after eating; he is fearful, especially at night. Our search narrows still more; then he adds the most enlightening symptom yet related: it seems as if there was a choking sensation rising up from his stomach into his throat and suffocating him, which brings on the attack. There are but two remedies to be thought of with this symptom, *Sepia* and *Mancinella*. The provings of *Mancinella* have brought out this symptom phrased by the provers exactly as the patient described it, while *Sepia* has a close counterpart. A comparison of the two remedies in relationship to the totality of the symptoms leaves us in no doubt but that the remedy is *Mancinella*.

Bœnninghausen once offered a prize for a " treatise concerning the greater or lesser (characteristic) value of the symptoms occurring in a disease, to aid as a norm or basis in the therapeutical selection of the remedy ". After three years of silence on the part of the homœopathic world, Bœnninghausen himself attempted to give what he considered a somewhat adequate answer. His reply was founded on Hahnemann's instructions in Paragraph 153 of the fifth edition of the *Organon* ; or, as Bœnninghausen puts it, this paragraph " contains the proper, true kernel of the answer . . . and deserves to be first premised ".

In seeking for the specific homœopathic remedy, i.e. in this juxtaposition of the phenomena of the natural disease and the list of the symptoms of the medicines, in order to discover a morbid potency corresponding in similitude to the evil to be cured, the more striking, particular, unusual and peculiar (characteristic) signs and symptoms of the case should be especially and almost solely kept in view ; for there must especially be some symptoms in the list of the medicine sought for corresponding to this, if the remedy should be the one most suitable to effect the cure. The more general and indefinite symptoms, such as lack of appetite, headache, weariness, disturbed sleep, uncomfortableness, etc., in their generalness and undefinedness deserve but little attention, unless they are more especially pronounced as something of a general nature is seen in almost every disease and in almost every medicine.

After this quotation from the *Organon*, Bœnninghausen continues :

It is seen, however, that it is here left to the physician to judge what is understood by the *more striking, particular, unusual and peculiar* symptoms, and it might, indeed, be difficult to furnish a commentary to this definition, which would not be too diffuse and therefore easily understood, and on the other hand would be complete enough to be properly applied to all these cases. . .

It is obvious that Hahnemann never intended his directions to be taken that we do keynote prescribing ; while his instructions were not to give undue weight to the most general of symptoms, it is to be remembered that Hahnemann never slighted any symptoms of a case in making a prescription. He had the genius of giving each symptom its true place in the picture without distorting the totality. While it is inconceivable that Hahnemann ever did keynote prescribing, it is also beyond our knowledge of Hahnemann's thorough mind that he eliminated the chief complaints in building up the symptom-image.

Our way, too, must lie in the golden mean between these two points, the one too general and the other too individual to assure us of a true totality. If we can find a remedy that has the " more striking, particular, unusual and peculiar (characteristic) signs and symptoms of the case " and in addition covers the chief complaint as well, we may consider ourselves as having a sound basis for the prescription of the *simillimum*

CHAPTER XII

THE DYNAMIC ACTION OF DRUGS

WE often speak of Hahnemann as the first to note the similar action of drugs and disease conditions, but history shows us that this is not so. Ten centuries B.C., the ancient Hindu system of medicine was founded on the theorem which, translated, reads in almost identical words to those Hahnemann used. Again, Aristotle, about 350 B.C., gave the following dictum :

If *simile* acts upon *simile*, the result of this mutual action reveals itself in neutralization, annihilation of the original qualities and in production of another state, which is exactly contrary to the previous one. . . . If the *simile* of the remedy acts upon the *simile* of the disease, the result of this mutual action is neutralization, annihilation of the original qualities, viz. of the pathopoiesis of the remedy and of the pathogenesis of the organism, and change into the contrary state, viz. health.

However it may be about the length of time elapsed since the recognition of the law of similars, the question of dose was one which Hahnemann solved.

The question of dose rests upon the philosophy pertaining to the practice of homœopathy. Ignoring the law of dosage reveals a lack of concept of the dynamic influence over matter. In life the dynamic force is the manifestation of life itself ; the body and tissues are not life, but they are the channels through which life functions.

The man who sees this glimpses the basis of vitalism ; that there is a whole world of causes prior to the world of effects ; that matter is indestructible and that force is transmitted through matter and therefore it, too, is indestructible. Matter may change in form but it is always present ; force may change its expression but no unit of force is ever destroyed. We hold that force, or energy, or dynamis, whatever you wish to call it, is *the law of nature* ;

it may express its power in different ways but in its essence it is that which was breathed into man at his creation which made him a living soul. The expression of this law may vary and find different expressions, as attraction, gravity, electricity, chemical affinity, dynamis, or spiritual power ; it is an expression of, and all combined under, one Head and Source of Power—God.

Hahnemann was a representative of this school of thought and he plumbed deeply into these mysteries. He became dissatisfied with the thought of his day, and read extensively the medical works of the ancients. In his delvings he found several, not long before his own time, like Stahl of Denmark and Halle of Switzerland, who had observed that medicines might cure disease by the power they possessed of causing like diseases in healthy human beings. He comprehended that these men had observed this phenomenon but that it had been allowed to fall into disuse without application. At this stage Hahnemann determined to discover the action of drugs upon human beings by observing all the details of their action upon healthy subjects.

Hahnemann did not originate this idea of proving drugs upon healthy individuals, but he was the first to so prove with a definite object in view. After thorough, painstaking, intelligent, systematic study and comparisons, after many long, tedious, self-sacrificing ordeals, Hahnemann was able to work out and announce to the world the existence of an heretofore unsuspected universal law of cure—not an occasional means of cure as had been anticipated by those of recent generations. This was the first step which culminated in the evolution of a new rational and scientific system of medical practice.

The full recognition of the law of similars rapidly succeeded the proving of drugs, and was the second step in the evolution of homœopathic principles.

Hahnemann began the experiments of the application of proven drugs for the cure of the sick upon the basis of the law of similars, by using drugs in their full strength. He found that many times the patient became greatly aggravated. Hahnemann reasoned that the dose was too large, and he experimented by diluting the drug on a definite scale ; to his surprise he found he secured better results. He continued this process until he discovered that the curative power of drugs bore no proportionate relationship to the crude quantity, but that under the peculiar and systematic reduction by a regular scale, and the proper manipulation, many drugs in common use, and many substances supposed to be inert in their crude states, became endowed with new and hitherto unsuspected activities and powers.

So Hahnemann, setting out simply to reduce the quantity of his doses, discovered potentization, an entirely new principle in posology, a wonderful development in the world of therapeutics, without which the law of cure would have been forgotten. This is the principle which gives life and power to the system of medicine which Hahnemann developed and this is the third great step in the evolution of the law of cure.

As Morgan says :

To Hahnemann alone is due imperishable honour and renown for discovering, first, the existence of an universal law of cure ; and second, that the specific properties of drugs could be developed, transmitted and utilized by potentization.

With the discovery of potentization, or dynamization, began the first practical tests of the newly-discovered law of cure.

Crude drugs have three grades of action : mechanical, chemical, and dynamic. The first two grades are of little comparative note in homœopathy. This is demonstrated by the fact that their provings in crude form produce comparatively little of worth, whereas in those provings made from the thirtieth and above we obtain more complete provings because of the dynamic action. The full power of the drug in its dynamic action is brought out in the potency, whereas the grosser material elements by their very crudity develop no fine individualities in their provings. Entirely new activities are developed, liberated, and may be transmitted and changed into the potentizing medium. (Cf. *Organon* 269.) This is shown by the potentization of inert substances like *Carbo veg.*, *Lycopodium* and *Silica*.

Let us look at a recent book (published 1933) dealing with

The Mode of Action of Drugs on Cells, by A. J. Clark, A.B., M.D., F.R.C.P., F.R.S., Professor of Materia Medica at the University of Edinburgh, formerly Professor of Pharmacology in the Universities of London and Cape Town. This book deals with the matter entirely from the orthodox medical viewpoint, yet hear his comment relative to the biological response of cell-drug reactions :

There is indeed very little direct evidence that the biological response is produced by a chemical reaction between the drug and the cell constituents. This assumption is chiefly justified by the facts that it is supported by much *indirect* evidence, and that there is no alternative hypothesis which has stronger evidence in its support. If we assume that there is some simple relation between the amount of drug entering into combination and the extent of the biological response, then the following consideration must apply.

If the fundamental chemical reaction consists in fixation of the drug by some particular constituent of the cell, then this must result in a reduction both of the free drug and of the free receptors in the cell. The relative amounts of drug solution and cells can, however, be varied at will, and hence the concentration of the drug can always be kept constant by providing a sufficient excess of drug solution ; indeed, in many cases *the quantity of the drug fixed is so minute that it is difficult to reduce the drug solution to a volume small enough to show changes of concentration* (p. 60).

Drugs that act in high dilutions are of particular interest in pharmacology, and in such cases true adsorption may be delayed by the depletion of the layer adjoining the surface. Freundlich (1926) states : " The simpler the conditions chosen and the smaller the difficulty in securing access to the inner surface, the quicker is the adsorption. . . . *In the case of well powdered adsorbments the equilibrium is mostly reached in seconds or minutes.* "

In the case of cell-drug solution systems in which vigorous stirring is possible . . . delay ought to be reduced. It is, however, necessary to remember that particles above a certain size carry with them a layer of water several micra thick, even when they are stirred thoroughly. Hence even in cases where such stirring is possible the delay due to depletion cannot be ignored. . . . (pp. 68-9).

In other words, even modern pharmacology recognizes
1. The reaction of amounts of drugs so minute that it is not

possible to tell how small the amount of the drug in the solution is, yet it still shows definite action on the cells. 2. The action is much more rapid in the case of well powdered substances (triturations). 3. Regardless of the quantity of the drug used, the solution is activated to a marked degree by vigorous stirring (succussion).

This shows the observations of the action of infinitesimal amounts of drug on the physiological basis, that the greater the trituration the more rapid the action, and that the influence of succussion also speeds the rate of activity markedly; but the comprehension of the vital principles upon which homœopathy is based does not follow the observations remarked by Professor Clark.

It is but natural that many prescribers at first stay close to the mechanical and chemical stages, for the material always first attracts our attention ; but in order to grasp this truth of dynamization we must apply the same means of approach and travel the same road that Hahnemann and his followers have travelled, recognizing the dynamic in health and in disease and applying the same line of thought and reason to the study and development of the power and action of drugs.

It is well to note the care and thoroughness of Hahnemann's work and the methodical way in which he developed the potency, using the centesimal scale in preparing his divided dosage, and giving each step in the process vigorous succussion. This process was continued until all trace of quantity had vanished, beyond the recognition of all possible physical tests ; yet in these higher potencies the dynamic qualities or potential qualities survive. Upon applying these potencies upon man or animals we find a far more delicate organism or apparatus than is provided in any possible physical instruments as yet developed. Possibly the furthest development of the radioactive power may in time give us a measuring instrument that may partially reveal this ability, but the human organism will always be the most delicate instrument, for the susceptible subject is quick to respond to this dynamic force.

We are dealing here in the realm of the imponderables,

and encounter problems beyond the reach of men's analysis, a realm where we can only observe effects alone. However, all we can see and all we can hope to know in our observation of human beings is the effects of growth and development ; and it is so with our study of medicinal action. This is so not only in the study of the potency, but it is so almost entirely in the study of the crude drugs and their action, as well as our study of foods and their action ; the effects are there to be seen, but the imponderable nature of the *modus operandi* is beyond our comprehension. The very same line of evidence is produced in all these fields ; it is the effects only that are manifest to us. The observations must be recorded, and only by deduction can we comprehend their innermost meaning. Many mistakes have been made by failing to follow rules laid down by Hahnemann in his *Organon of the Healing Art*. Follow these rules and the results will be in order and observable.

Many of the graduates from homœopathic colleges do not grasp the dynamic concept of drugs, and for that reason always stay in the material plane, using only the crude drug or venturing into the low potencies occasionally. This is unfortunate for the efficacy of their work, for once this concept is grasped they realize that all potencies are valuable and useful, and they soon obtain a knowledge and power over disease little realized when viewed solely from the material plane. Especially is this true in chronic troubles, for the test of real skill is in the cure of chronic patients and the eradication of the chronic miasms.

The use of the attenuated potency varies with each individual because of his interpretation of the law of dose. Hahnemann's question as to " how far the dose of a homœopathic remedy in any given case of disease ought to be reduced in order to derive from it the best possible cure ? " is one we may well ask.

It may be readily conceived that no theoretical conjecture will furnish an answer to this problem, and it is not by such means that we can establish, in respect to each individual medicine, the quantity of the dose that suffices to produce the homœopathic effect and accomplish a prompt and gentle cure. No reasoning, however ingenious, will avail in this instance. It is by pure experiments and precise observations only that this object can be obtained.

Organon, 278. Here the question arises, as to the proper degree of reduction at which a medicine will procure certain as well as gentle relief? That is to say, how small must be the dose of each homœopathically selected medicine, in order to fulfil the requirement of a perfect cure. To determine the dose of each particular medicine for this purpose, and how to render this dose so small as to accomplish its purpose gently and rapidly at the same time, is a problem which, obviously, is neither to be solved by theoretical conjecture, nor by sophistic reasoning. Pure experiments, and accurate observation alone can solve the question ; and it were folly to adduce the large doses of the old school (destitute of homœopathic bearing upon the diseased portion of the body, and affecting only the sound parts), to disprove the results of actual experience in regard to the minuteness of doses requisite to perform a homœopathic cure.

279. Experience proves that *the dose of a homœopathically selected remedy cannot be reduced so far as to be inferior in strength to the natural disease, and to lose its power of extinguishing and curing at least a portion of the same, provided that this dose, immediately after having been taken, is capable of causing a slight intensification of symptoms of the similar natural disease* (slight homœopathic aggravation, 157-160). This will prove to be the case in acute, chronic, and even complicated diseases, except where these depend on serious deterioration of some vital organ, or where the patient is not protected against extraneous medicinal influences.

280. This incontrovertible principle, founded on experience, furnishes a standard *according to which the doses of homœopathic medicine are invariably to be reduced so far, that even after having been taken, they will merely produce an almost imperceptible homœopathic aggravation.* We should not be deterred from the use of such doses by the high degree of rarefaction that may have been reached, however incredible they may appear to the coarse material ideas of ordinary practitioners ; their arguments will be silenced by the verdict of infallible experience.

Since Hahnemann's time potentization has been greatly developed, and we are often able to avoid these slight aggravations which Hahnemann refers to as almost a necessary accompaniment to the cure. When we get these aggravations now it is because the remedy has been given too low or repeated too often, or because the patient is particularly susceptible to the powers released by the potentization. When this slight aggravation of the natural disease appears after the administration of the remedy it is an indication of the correct choice of the remedy.

All authorities agree that the proper dose is found in the degree of susceptibility. Fincke says, " That dose is appropriate which will be proportionate to the degree of susceptibility of the patient."

The closer the relationship between the disease symptoms and the drug symptoms, the greater the susceptibility and, consequently, the higher the potency required ; but this makes it a comparative problem of relationship ; therefore the answer lies in our individual exercise of the interpretation of this law.

It is a hopeful sign when the younger physicians begin with the use of the fairly low potencies, say the 30th or 200th, and then progress upward. In this way one learns for himself the use of potencies and their dynamic action, and he will soon learn to use the higher potencies with skill and with much satisfaction.

Fincke explained the action and efficiency of the infinitesimal dose by applying the law of Maupertius, the French mathematician, and fully accepted by scientists, " that the quantity of action necessary to effect any change in nature is the least possible " ; and added, " according to this principle the decisive moment is always a minimum, an infinitesimal ", and when applied to therapeutics the last possible or the highest potency, sufficient to bring about reaction, would be homœopathic.

The law of least action is a necessary complement to the law of similars. Still quoting Fincke,

According to this principle, the curative properties and action of the homœopathic remedy are governed by its preparation and application ; in other words, *the quality of the action of a homœopathic remedy is determined by its quantity*, consequently the law of the least action must be acknowledged as the posological principle of homœopathy.

The whole range of potencies may be used by any

physician, yet if he understands these principles he will feel his way to the correct potency. There is no greater fallacy prevalent than the fear of using the higher potencies, for fear the lower would be more effective ; the same indications are present for one as for the other.

The knowledge of potentization was of gradual growth, and, indeed, the last word is not yet said ; but this discovery ranks among the highest of Hahnemann's work and makes the question of the use of these potencies the one great thing that is due to Hahnemann's mind alone, and will be his greatest lasting contribution in the evolution of this system of applying drugs to the cure of disease.

It has remained so far unexplainable, but a fact. The effect is manifest to all, but in its mode of action it is a mystery. The principle of similars was of little practical use until the principle of the dynamic use of drugs and the minimum dose were discovered to complete the trinity ; then all three angles were complete, each equally important, yet each supporting the other to make a complete system of cure ; then, and only then, homœopathy became practicable.

Were it not for the knowledge of the dynamis of drugs and the minimum dose, homœopathy would have sunk back with the memory of Hahnemann's provings of a few drugs, as it did after the work of Hippocrates, Haller, and Stahl. This is where the great genius of Hahnemann shines forth and will continue to shed lustre more and more as time goes on.

The discovery and development of the dynamic principle in medicine was a forerunner of the knowledge of many things that are generally accepted by the scientific world although they remain among " the things hard to be understood ". Our wonderful development in electricity, with the radioactivity of matter, the radio, chemical affinity, and many other scientific discoveries have been made possible as similar, almost parallel, discoveries to this of Hahnemann. It was the direct cause of the rejection of Newton's concept of matter as a " hard, massy, material atom ", and passing on to the acceptance of the concept of the electron and our present-day concept of the minuteness of matter ; and it will eventually force the recognition of the infinite divisibility and the fourth dimension of matter.

The power developed by the process of dynamis is tremendous when it can take solid substances and make them tremendously useful in medicine. It is nothing less than a physical process by which the dynamic energy, latent in crude substances, is liberated, developed, and modified for use in medicine. The true dynamic action and principle was bound to be imitated in the attempt to modify violent poisonous morbific products of disease by transmitting them through living animals and so make them of use in medicine. The serums are an attempt in a crude way to imitate the simple though correct method of releasing power from violent poisons, but it is very inaccurate in principle, for living animals are constantly varying in many degrees, and it is fraught with many uncertainties. Stuart Close has well compared this process in enunciating the standards of Hahnemann :

1. The Hahnemannian process is purely physical, objective and mechanical.

2. It does not involve any uncertain, unseen, unreliable nor unmeasurable factor. Its elements are simply the substance or drug to be potentiated, a vehicle consisting of sugar of milk, alcohol or water, in certain quantities and definite proportions ; manipulation under conditions which are entirely under control and so simple that a child could comply with them.

3. The resulting product is stable, or may easily be made so ; in fact, it is almost indestructible ; and the experience of a century, in its use under homœopathic methods and principles had proved it to be efficient and reliable in the treatment of all forms of disease amenable to medication.

4. The process is practically illimitable. Potentiation of medicine by this method may be carried to any extent desired or required.

The experience of the practicable application of this power in disease is the final test and arbiter of their power, and it always proves their value as the correct process in the cure of the sick ; yet even after repeated experience we cannot fail to marvel at the universe of latent power released by so simple a method. Again quoting from Stuart Close :

The fact, as pointed out by Ozanam, is that Hahnemann, by his discovery of potentiation, raised homœopathy to a level with other natural sciences, since he created for it a method which is analogous to the infinitesimal calculus of mathematics, upon which is based the atomic theory of chemistry. It illustrates and harmonizes with the " theory of the interatomic ether of space "; the " theory of the radiant state of matter "; the theory of the electric potential of present-day physics, and with the chemico-cellular theory of physiology and pathological anatomy. It agrees with modern bacteriology in its explanation of the action of pathogenic micro-organisms as being due to the infinitesimal quantities of their secreted poisons. It is in harmony with the latest conclusions of modern psychology.

What is the relation between dynamis and the homœopathic dosage ?

What was the first step in the evolution of homœopathic therapeutics ?   (*Answer :* Drug proving.)

What was the second step ?   (*Answer :* Discovery of the law of similars.)

What was the third step ?   (*Answer :* The principle of potentiation.)

What is the benefit of potentizing so-called inert substances ?

Give an outline of the method of potentizing drugs as laid down by Hahnemann.

Differentiate *dilution* and *potentization*.

Explain the application of the law of mathematics to the homœopathic principles of the action of potentized drugs.

How does the law of least action referred to, answer Hahnemann's questions as to how far the dose of a homœopathic remedy . . . ought to be reduced in order to derive from it the best possible cure ?

Give three reasons which may account for an aggravation of the symptoms after the administration of the remedy.

Why do we find the greater the susceptibility the higher the potency required ?   (Cf. Law of least action.)

CHAPTER XIII

THE DOSE

IN considering the amount of medicine to be used at one time, or to answer the query, What constitutes a dose ? it is very important to have some concept of the history of homœopathy, for this throws light upon the development of the problem of dosage.

Before Hahnemann's time, and indeed in his early work, the dose played an important part. Nothing but crude and massive doses had ever been used in the care of the sick. All physicians used these massive doses as a matter of course, and Hahnemann, being a product of the best training of that day, followed, in his early career, in the footsteps of his predecessors. Even after Hahnemann began to see the light of the LAW OF CURE he continued to use massive doses, and it is to be remembered that he made cures with massive doses of crude medicine, but from his close observations and continual experiments he found that he was obtaining drug effects oftener than he was making a successful cure.

When he became convinced of this, he reduced the dose, dividing and again dividing the dose, watching closely the results. He soon found that the smaller the dose, the more beneficent the results. His experiments with the divided dose did not come until after he had discovered the dynamic action of disease ; then with his logical mind he must of necessity have correlated his results from the larger doses and brought his ideas of dosage into correlation with the same concept. For if disease be dynamic in nature, the use of a remedy to cure, or even to reach the disease, must be dynamic, rather than physiological, in form and power.

The more Hahnemann became convinced of the dynamic nature of disease, the more he sought the dynamic plane in medicine, and the more beneficial he found the administration of the similia. Very, very gradually, the minimum dose, which is always a flexible measure, became ever smaller and smaller, until it has developed into the infinitesimal.

However, it has been a long road to the use of the minimum dose, and many animosities have developed, all because of the failure of many minds to grasp the idea of the dynamic nature of disease and the natural tendency to look upon material substance as the remedy and the pathological state as the disease, and the failure to see the expression of diseased states in subjective symptoms.

The gradual recognition of the power of the minimum dose is manifest even in the dominant school of medicine, and is being proven in the laboratories of modern science. As a result, gradually lessening doses are being adopted by many who have formerly derided the possibility of effectiveness from small doses. Many of the leading pharmacies have followed this road in preparing drugs for the use of the general physician. This trend is manifest in the colloidal preparations and the ductless gland therapy. Of late the physiologist has shown the power of vitamins, and as a particular instance we might point to recent experiments with Vitamin D. It has been found that one part of the crystalline form to three-trillionths has a curative action on rachitis, while one part to fifty-thousandths has a destructive action to the point of causing rickets. This again verifies Hahnemann's dictum on the power of the small dose and the harmful effects of the more material dosage, although this proven material would be classed as infinitesimal by many.

This also demonstrates the Arndt-Schulz law of action and reaction. So we are coming to a point where we fully recognize and comprehend the soundness of Hahnemann's deductions. Let us go to Hahnemann's *Organon* (fifth American edition) for his teaching in regard to the dose, remembering that in every edition this was plainly taught. Each edition progressed one step further in the development of the minuteness of the dose.

Paragraph 112. In older descriptions of the fatal effects of overdoses of medicines, it is often to be noticed that the close of such deplorable accidents was marked by certain effects which were of very different nature from those witnessed at the beginning of the case. These symptoms which are called forth in opposition to the primary effect, or actual operation of drugs upon the vital force of the organism, are its counter-effect, or after-effect. But these are rarely if ever perceived after moderate doses administered to healthy persons for the purpose of experiment ; and they are altogether absent after minute doses. During the homœopathic curative process, the living organism exhibits only that degree of counteraction against these minute doses, which is required to re-establish the natural state of health.

128. The most recent experiments have taught that crude medicinal substances . . . will not disclose the same wealth of latent powers as when they are taken in a highly attenuated state, potentiated by means of trituration and succusion. Through this simple process the powers hidden and dormant, as it were, in the crude drug, are developed, and called into activity in an incredible degree.

156. There is, however, scarcely a homœopathic remedy which, though well selected, if not sufficiently reduced in its dose, might not call forth at least one unusual sensation, or slight new symptom during its operation on very susceptible and sensitive patients. . . .

157. Although a homœopathically selected remedy, by virtue of its fitness and minuteness of dose, quietly cancels or extinguishes an analogous disease. . . . Aggravation caused by larger doses may last for several hours, but in reality these are only drug-effects somewhat superior in intensity, and very similar to the original disease.

159. The smaller the dose of the homœopathic remedy, so much the smaller and shorter is the apparent aggravation of the disease during the first hours.

160. The dose of a homœopathic remedy can scarcely be reduced to such a degree of minuteness as to make it powerless to overcome, and to completely cure an analogous, natural disease of recent origin, and undisturbed by injudicious treatment. We may, therefore, readily understand why a less minute dose of a suitable homœopathic medicine, an hour after its exhibition, may produce an appreciable, homœopathic aggravation of this kind.

In Hahnemann's *Chronic Diseases* he is equally emphatic when he says :

But when these aggravated original symptoms appear later on in the same strength as at the beginning, or even more strongly later on, this is a sign that the dose of this antipsoric remedy although it was correctly selected, was too great, and caused the fear that no cure could be effected through it, since medicines given in so large a dose are able to establish a disease which in some respects is similar, but even greater and more troublesome, without extinguishing the old disease. This is caused by the fact that the medicine used in so large a dose unfolds also its other symptoms which nullify its similarity and thus establishes another dissimilar disease, also chronic, in place of the former.

Again he says :

This (the large dose of medicine) finds its decision already in the first sixteen, eighteen or twenty days of the effect of the medicine given in too large a dose, as it must then be checked, either by prescribing its antidote, or when this is not known, by giving another antipsoric medicine, as suitable as possible to the symptoms then prevailing, and this in a very moderate dose, and when this is not yet sufficient for abolishing this sinister medicinal disease by prescribing a second medicine as suitable as possible at that time. . . . When the stormy assault of the excessive dose of even a correctly selected homœopathic remedy has been assuaged by the following use of an antidote or the later use of some other antipsoric remedy, this remedy which had only proved injurious through its excessive strength may be used again, and indeed as it is homœopathically indicated with the best success, only in a far smaller dose and in a far more highly potentized attenuation.

And still again :

No harm will be done if the dose given is even smaller than I have indicated. It can hardly be too small if only everything is avoided that might interfere with the action of the medicine or obstruct it. . . . They will even then do everything of good that can in general be expected of medicine, if only the antipsoric was selected correctly in all respects as to the carefully examined symptoms of the disease and was thus homœopathic, and the patient did not by his actions disturb the medicine in its action. . . . On the other hand, we have the great advantage that even if in some case the selection should not have been made quite suitably, we have the great advantage that we can easily put out of action the wrong medicine in its minimal dose in the manner indicated above, when the treatment can be continued with a suitable antipsoric without delay.

If prescribers in general, and especially those starting on the path of homoeopathic prescribing, would take special note of this warning, they would save themselves much trouble and their patients much needless suffering. Hahnemann felt the waste of time, effort, and actual suffering needlessly caused, when he cried :

What would they have risked if they had at once heeded my words and had first made use of these small doses ? Could anything worse have happened than that these small doses might have proved ineffectual ? They could not have injured anybody ! But in their unintelligent self-willed use of large doses in homoeopathic practice they only passed again through the same roundabout route, so dangerous to their patients, which I in order to save them the trouble had already passed through with trembling, but successfully, and after doing much mischief and having wasted much time they had eventually if they wanted to cure to arrive at the only correct goal, which I had made known to them long before faithfully and openly, giving to them the reasons therefor.

That Boenninghausen also passed through this "roundabout route" is witnessed by his words in his *Lesser Writings*, quoting from an earlier statement in *Homoeopathy, a Reader for the Cultivated, Non-medical Public* : "Since I also, led by the almost unanimous assertions as to the untenableness of this teaching, gave, though only for a short time, larger doses and with bad success."

Homoeopathic dosage is based upon law, as is the selection of the remedy based upon the law of similars. ACTION AND REACTION ARE EQUAL AND OPPOSITE : this is fundamental, and it is this law that must guide us in the application of drugs.

The so-called primary action of drugs, and the so-called secondary action of drugs, are manifest to any observer. As a common illustration we may take the nausea and vomiting of *Ipecacuhana* ; yet in small doses it is curative in sickness with nausea and vomiting as prominent symptoms, other symptoms agreeing. *Opium* causes profound sleep when used in the ordinary manner ; yet *Opium* is of inestimable value when given homoeopathically, in small doses, in cases of profound coma. These instances cited are of drugs

classic in massive doses, or, in common parlance, physiological doses, for certain common states of sickness.

The physiological action of a drug, however, has nothing
whatever to do with the curative action from the homœopathic point of view, because homœopathic remedies are
never used in physiological doses. This may seem at first
illogical because we may use them in low potencies, yet we
never use them for their physiological effect.

The physiological action is toxic in nature, therefore
injurious to the patient. The physiological action of a drug
is not its therapeutic or curative action ; it is the exact
opposite of a curative action and is never employed in
homœopathic practice for curative effects. The use of the
drug in physiological form is an acknowledgment of the
attempt to produce drug symptoms because of their primary
action, and an acknowledgment also that the physician so
using the drug has never observed the secondary symptoms.
Speaking of narcotic drugs, in Paragraph 113 of his *Organon*,
Hahnemann has this to say :

. . . As these (narcotic drugs) destroy sensibility and
sensation, as well as irritability, in their primary effect, a
heightened state both of sensibility and irritability is frequently
observed in healthy persons, as an after-effect following the
administration of narcotics, even in moderate doses.

Pathogenetic is the term used by the homœopathicians as
a more correct term for the primary symptoms produced by
the drug, and as a synonym for the term *toxic* ; in other
words symptoms may be produced by massive doses or by
crude drugs, but these symptoms are pathogenetic and not
curative. These symptoms may show forth family likenesses
as many members of a family, under certain circumstances,
will often have a similar general reaction ; but to apply our
knowledge of the drug as a curative measure we must know
definitely what its capabilities are. These capabilities
cannot be manifest from the pathogenetic symptoms.

The homœopathic cure is produced without drug effects ;
it is accomplished without suffering ; it is mild ; it is developed through growth ; it is dynamic in nature, therefore it
must be given on the dynamic plane and never in a way to

produce drug effects. It therefore must be the minimum amount of the drug that will act upon the vital force, which, as Hahnemann says, can scarcely be too small.

We must remember, in the dividing of the dose, no matter how far this is extended there is something of the drug left. Matter is never destroyed ; it may be changed in potentization, but an absolute zero is never reached.

Homœopathic dosages require that no new symptoms shall be produced as a result of their administration, for these would be drug effects ; but we may find a slight aggravation of the symptoms already present immediately following the administration of the homœopathic remedy, which soon recedes, and improvement continues. Only the single remedy in the smallest possible dose will usher in these happy results in this way ; the suffering is quickly reduced ; the strength is conserved ; the patient is in a state of restored health.

We must not think that the infinitesimal dose cannot produce symptoms ; this is frequently found in very susceptible patients. In fact, the best provings are obtained with the high potencies on susceptible people.

When the homœopathic drug is administered, it is so similar to the natural disease that it therefore meets with no resistance, because the sphere of its action is already invaded by the similar disease and its resistance overcome by the similar acting disease-producing agent. The affected organs and tissues are open to attack ; susceptibility to the similar remedy is therefore greatly increased. The homœopathic remedy acts upon the identical tracts involved in disease states in a similar way to the disease-producing cause. In order that the suffering and distress may not be increased, it is therefore necessary to use only the smallest possible dose. For this reason the homœopathic dose is always short of the physiological or pathogenetic dose. It must be so small as not to produce too much aggravation of the symptoms already present, and never large enough to produce new symptoms.

There is a law of dosage as well as a law of cure, and when we use a homœopathic remedy it should be based upon that law, for if homœopathy means anything, it is that it is based upon natural law and order. This law is fixed and unchangeable. It makes no difference with the law if we do not follow it, but it does make a difference with our results. *The quantity of action necessary to effect any change in nature is the least possible : the decisive amount is always a minimum, an infinitesimal.*

It can hardly fail to be plain that the same power which establishes the curative relationship between drugs and diseases, and regulates this law, should at the same time and in the same manner determine the quantity and method of this administration. This places it, not upon a notion or whim of what strength shall be used, but upon our interpretation of the law.

Let us elucidate this law. Let us get a clear concept of the elements of this problem. They are of two classes : those which belong to the patient, and those which are associated with the drug.

In the first, we are dealing with the perverted stimulus of the organs or functions of the body and the natural relationships are disturbed. The susceptibility of these organs to impressions from these stimuli are exalted, depressed, or extinguished. The susceptibility may be exalted in respect to some influences even to the point of intolerance, or depressed in others to the point where we have the feeblest response to impressions, while others are entirely void of response to all stimuli. These are new susceptibilities to impressions from external forces not found at all, or not existing to the same degree, in the healthy. The sum of these changes forms a class of facts most important in this investigation, and gives the basis of a proper understanding of the condition of the sick.

For our present purpose it will be necessary to consider only such of these changes as have reference to impressions from drugs. In a given case of disease the patient is often over-sensitive to the smallest quantity of some drugs, while there is an equal insensibility to even large quantities of others. We find this often. The answer to this is an illustration of the expression of the law of the dose. The changes of susceptibility constitute the first class of the general elements of the problem. Those of the second belong to the drug.

These consist of the power which belongs to drugs to produce disturbances in the action of living forces, so that they no longer act in harmony which maintains that sense of well-being which is health. It is this power so to act that constitutes a drug, and it is with this power so to act upon living organs in special conditions of susceptibility that we have to do in determining the dose in a given case of disease and also to comprehend as the law which governs the dose in all cases.

After having settled the first question in prescribing— What is the remedy ?—this question of special susceptibility in the organs is just that which decides the next question we must answer : How much of this remedy is required to restore the lost balance of the vital force in the particular case ? In these two questions lies the whole problem of cure.

How can we know the degree of the special susceptibility to the action of the drug before its administration ? Simply by the same process of inquiry that led to the choice of the true remedy ; it is that which is *like* ; it is what the drug, whose action on the healthy living organism is most like the phenomena of the lost balance of the vital energy which we call disease. Then institute this inquiry : *How much is it like ?* This answer determines the quantity of the drug required, and *this is in the inverse ratio of the similarity.* This constitutes the basic law of the dose as to quantity and potency.

What is the like, the similarity ? The like which cures is the resemblance of the characteristic symptoms of the drug to those of the disease ; the characteristic symptoms of the disease and the drug are those symptoms that give to each its individual character, *not* all those symptoms held in common with the general disease group or the family group of drugs.

It is the similarity of the characteristic symptoms of the drug to those of the disease ; and again, how nearly similar it is to the number of characteristic symptoms, that marks the exact similitude. The greater the number of characteristic symptoms of the disease that are found to correspond to the drug, the less the quantity and the higher the potency that can be used.

The whole relationship of drugs to disease rests on the susceptibility. The power of the drug over disease is solely in its similarity ; without it, it has no power except in a physiological form, and that is never curative. If in the patient there be wanting a susceptibility to its impressions, this relationship of the patient to the drug does not exist. It rests on the very similarity of those elements of the disease which show its specific nature, to those which are characteristic of the drug and according to the degree of susceptibility ; it is in direct ratio to this susceptibility.

In sickness, susceptibility is markedly increased, as the avenues of diseased states are widely opened so that which would have no effect in health will be quickly grasped in disease. The resemblance of the group of symptoms is marked, therefore accordingly the very smallest possible dose will satisfy the susceptibility and therefore be curative.

A knowledge of the basic principles of this law explains why often a very high potency will cure intractable disease states where the low potencies do not even give relief. Again, the knowledge of this law necessitates a thorough knowledge of our materia medica. A knowledge of this law makes for a clearer understanding of the homœopathic art.

Why did Hahnemann first begin to experiment with the divided dose ?

Why do we believe that the remedy should be dynamic in action ?

What did Hahnemann mean when he said : " . . . crude medicinal substances . . . will not disclose the same wealth of latent powers as when they are taken in a highly attenuated state " ?

What is the simple process that liberates the latent powers in the diluted substances ?

What is a homœopathic aggravation of a disease ?

What symptoms are produced by massive doses or crude drugs ?

Why are these symptoms of little or no value in homœopathic prescribing ?

Why do we believe that the law of least action is that which should be our law of dosage ?

What two elements enter into our consideration of the cure of disease conditions ?

What relation does the degree of similarity of drug symptoms to disease symptoms bear to the size of the dose ?

On what does the relationship of drugs to disease rest ? (*Answer* : Susceptibility.)

What effect does sickness have on the susceptibility of the patient ?

Why does this explain the efficiency of a high potency when a low potency does not give relief ?

CHAPTER XIV

REMEDY REACTION

ONE of the first things required of a homœopathic physician is that his powers of observation shall be highly developed. His powers of discrimination should be very keenly attuned, first, that he may observe the patient in the analysis of the symptoms and the selection of the remedy, and second, that he may have the keen perception of the import of the symptoms after the remedy has been carefully selected and administered. After the administration of the *simillimum* some action should result. It is upon the development and interpretation of the action of the remedy, or the reaction of the vital energy to the remedy, that successful prescribing very largely depends.

What are we to expect after the remedy has been administered ? According to Hahnemann, the nearer similar the remedy the more reaction we may expect (*Organon*, 154, 155). If the exact *simillimum* is found we are apt to get a slight aggravation before relief comes. On the other hand, if no changes take place, too long patient waiting is useless, for it is evidence that the *simillimum* has not been found ; but the nearer the symptoms of the patient are to the symptoms of the remedy, the more sure we are to have some reaction. It is for us to determine what the reaction means and to interpret it in prognostic terms. We must be able to listen to the patient's report and from it and our powers of observation to determine what the remedy is doing. We know that when the remedy acts the symptoms will change, in either character or degree. There may be a disappearance of the symptoms, amelioration of the symptoms or increase of the symptoms, and these changes are the manifest action of the remedy on the vital energy or vital force ; and it is these manifestations we must study.

Among the most common reactions after the remedy has been administered is aggravation or amelioration. Now there are two types of aggravations, either of which may be manifest. There is the aggravation which is an aggravation of the disease condition, in which the patient grows worse. There may be a very different type of aggravation, in which the symptoms are worse, but the patient is growing better. He will say, " I feel better, Doctor, but such-and-such symptoms are worse." The aggravation from the diseased state is an indication that the patient is growing weaker, and therefore the diseased state is growing stronger while his vital energy is ebbing. On the other hand, the aggravation of the symptoms while the patient reports himself as feeling better is an indication that his vital force is being set in order, but individual symptoms may show aggravation.

We must also observe how the aggravation or amelioration occurs and the duration of these periods. In this connection we must always bear in mind that it is the patient's welfare we are seeking, and it is for us to determine whether he is improving or declining. Sometimes he will say that he is weaker, yet on analysis of the symptoms you will find this is not true. The story of the symptoms is often of greater importance than the patient's opinion. After we have assured him of the amelioration of his condition and called his attention to the particular instances of improvement, he will feel better immediately.

The aggravation when the patient is growing actually weaker is a sure indication that the symptoms are taking on a more internal phase and the vital organs are more affected. In other words, it is an illustration of the reversal of the order of cure. In these states the patient may sometimes declare himself better, because of the absence of some trying symptoms, yet the careful homœopathic observer will know he is worse because the natural course of cure is reversed and the disease condition is attacking more vital parts. By these differentiations we know whether the patient is progressing or retrogressing. In many of these cases there is corroboration between the patient and the symptoms in the mind of the patient himself ; and just in so far as there is this corroboration, the truth of his observations is valuable. We should find whether the symptoms are tending toward the exterior and away from the inner parts. In other words we should know whether there is a peripheral tendency, or a tendency in the reverse order.

The aggravation of the diseased state may come from an incurable state which is stirred to its foundations by the potentized remedy, and unless the remedy is counteracted the disease will become worse and more rapidly approach a fatal termination. In borderline cases, cases bordering on fatal termination, the use of extremely high potencies may react on the vital energy so deeply as to cause an aggravation of the disease, whereas a more moderate potency (say the 30th or 200th) would not give such dangerously powerful effects. However, no fatal aggravation will occur unless it is already foreshadowed by the symptoms manifest in the patient. The potentized remedy will never produce a fatal aggravation, or a destructive aggravation, that would not have been possible and even probable from the symptomatology ; but it may, and often does, when used without discretion, speed the case to a fatal termination. In other words, a single dose of the high potency will not produce disease conditions ; it has the power to develop conditions that are already present if it is used carelessly or ignorantly. More careful study might reveal the indications for a less deeply acting remedy, which when administered would greatly mitigate much of the fatal suffering.

You must remember that we are warned in the *Organon* to discern what is curative in medicine, and also what is curable in disease. This point cannot be too greatly stressed : that in profound states we must be very careful not to stir the vital energy to its depths. There should be more time allowed for attempt at a gradual restoration, as there has likewise been a gradual decline. Very often less deeply acting remedies will react and palliate incurable diseases because they act more superficially. They act upon the sensorium and do not act upon the deep recesses of the vital force itself, and yet make the patient much more comfortable by relieving the symptoms annoying through the sensorium.

We can know, then, whether changes are occurring from the depths of the vital force or whether the patient may recover. The direction taken by the symptoms is the sure indication.

In this connection, the first observation is often a prolonged aggravation and a final decline of the patient. Now just what has happened ? Possibly there has been too deep an antipsoric administered and it has set in motion the vital energy and developed a destructive process. In these profound states of incurables the vital reaction toward cure is impossible and we can be assured that it is an incurable case. In such cases as these profound incurable conditions we should avoid giving a high potency of the remedy ; by administering a lower potency we may be able to go on and develop the case gradually until later it may possibly react favourably to a higher potency. This is well illustrated in advanced cases of tuberculosis, where it is never safe to give a very high attenuation of the exact *simillimum*. It is probably wiser not to use an antipsoric in these conditions. However, this applies only to those who are profoundly ill with chronic troubles.

In cases where there is not so profound a disturbance, after the remedy has been administered, the aggravation may be long and severe, yet the final reaction and amelioration comes. Sometimes in these states the aggravation may even last for weeks, yet improvement in general is continually taking place and then comes the amelioration and a slow but sure recovery, so that the second observation would be a long aggravation but final although slow improvement.

In these borderline cases there has already been established some marked organic changes, and where pathological changes have actually taken place the period of aggravation will be longer, but the general improvement in health in the curable cases will be manifest.

Then there is another reaction, where the aggravation is quick and short and strong, with rapid improvement of the patient. When you find such a reaction to the remedy you will always find rapid improvement. The reaction is vigorous and there has been no structural change of the vital organs. If there have been structural changes they have been of a superficial nature and near the surface and not of the vital parts, such manifestations as furunculosis or abscess formations on the surface. These are surface changes and are not comparable to the effects of the changes in the deeper organs, like the kidneys, the heart, or the brain.

It is well to take note of the difference between organic changes that take place in the vital organs that sustain the economy, which we cannot do without, and those that take place in less vital parts of the body and are not vital to life itself.

An aggravation that is quick, short, and strong is to be desired, because we know that improvement will be rapid.

Again, there is another class of indications where we find no aggravation whatsoever. There is no organic change ; there is no tendency to organic disease. The chronic condition causing disturbances to which the remedy is applicable is not of very great depth, it belongs to the functional conditions, exhibiting its effects in the nervous manifestations and the relations of the patient to his surroundings and to tissue changes. There are changes in the vital force that are so profound as to cause many symptoms that are very trying to the patient and yet so slight that with all the instruments of precision we do not observe any pathological changes. It is in these conditions that we sometimes get considerable suffering, yet cures will come without any aggravation. In these cases the single remedy in a moderate potency (say the 200th) will probably complete the work. In such cases we know the potency and the remedy are correct.

Then we have some cases with amelioration coming first and aggravation coming afterward. This amelioration comes on to last usually for three or four days ; the patient seems to be better but at the end of a week or ten days all the symptoms are worse than when he first came to you. These are usually cases that have a great many symptoms. We find that, in spite of what we thought at first was a favourable reaction, the ultimate condition is unfavourable. Either we selected too superficial a remedy, that could act only as a palliative, or the case is incurable and the remedy has been somewhat similar but not completely so. In order to determine the cause of the reaction we must examine the patient and find out whether the symptoms related to the remedy or to the disease. Sometimes you will find the remedy was in error. You will find usually in these cases that the remedy was similar to the most pronounced symptoms but it did not cover the whole case, and therefore did not strike at the constitutional state of the patient. Here in evaluating the symptoms we missed the essential concomitants, and we based our prescription on the generals only. It may be that we have an incurable patient. It will be fortunate for such cases if the symptoms come back exactly as they were when you first saw the case, but the symptoms often come back changed. Then we must wait, and this will require patience on the part of the physician and co-operation on the part of the patient. It may be necessary to take the patient into your confidence, if he evinces sufficient intelligence to warrant it.

The higher potencies will set in motion in the vital force curative functions which will act a long time, because oftentimes in these chronic conditions it takes a long time to establish order, and the vital energy takes its own time to cure. During this process no medicine should be given.

In cases that are proceeding to a perfect cure, if the improvement continues for some time and then suddenly comes to a halt, find out if the patient has been doing something that is against the rules of health or has interfered with the continuation of the curative action of the remedy. This will often be found to be the cause of too short a period of relief from the symptoms.

In the third observation you will remember there was a quick aggravation followed by a long amelioration. Note the difference here. You have just considered the amelioration, that was of too short duration. In instances where you have an aggravation immediately after the administration of the remedy, and then a quick rebound, you never see too short amelioration of the remedy. If there is a quick rebound, the amelioration should last. If it does not last, it is because of some condition that interferes with the action of the remedy. It may be something that the patient is doing entirely unconsciously, or it may be something that he is doing deliberately and intentionally. A quick rebound means everything to the case. It means that the remedy is well chosen, that it covers the condition of the vital economy ;

and if everything goes without interference, it will bring ultimate recovery.

There is this to remember : some remedies have an aggravation immediately after administration, and some have a sharp aggravation some little time after administration. For instance, *Phosphorus* may have a sharp aggravation, but it rarely occurs under twenty-four hours after administration, and it may be forty-eight hours or longer, and it may last for some little time.

A word about the acute cases in conditions where you get a quick rebound and amelioration lasting for a few hours, only to have another aggravation, when the action of the remedy on the vital force is exhausted. The action of the remedy is much more quickly exhausted in the rapid pace of acute diseases than in the more moderate progress of chronic manifestations, and more frequent repetitions of the remedy may be demanded. The most satisfactory amelioration in acute cases is where amelioration comes gradually and takes an hour or two after the administration of the remedy before it is markedly manifest.

If amelioration is too short in chronic diseases it means that structural changes are taking place and have destroyed or threatened to destroy the proper functions of the patient. It takes close observation to discern these changes from the reaction of the remedy. However, one may acquire much help from careful observation of these indications in detecting the course and progress of the case.

Once in a great while you will find a full period of amelioration of the symptoms, yet no special relief of the patient. This you will encounter in cases where you have structural changes, where the patient will improve on the remedy for some time and then improvement will cease. They can improve only to a certain point, and then improvement can go no further. We meet these conditions where organs like the liver or kidneys are partially involved and can function only in part. The remedy may keep the patient comfortable, however ; and by careful repetitions of the remedy at infrequent intervals the patient may be kept comfortable for a considerable period of time even though you will not be justified in expecting a cure.

There is another reaction that we find in some patients, and that is purely hysterical. They seem to prove any remedy you may give them and get an aggravation from it. This may be because of an idiosyncrasy for the remedy or because of too sensitive reaction of the vital energy. It may be almost impossible to do anything with them in a curative way, but it may be of inestimable help in proving a remedy. Before a remedy is used the constitutional condition of the patient should be very carefully noted. Write down the peculiarities of the patient in as much detail as possible, and then these observations should be deducted from the proving.

In a case where the symptoms found by careful questioning seem to be entirely adequate to cover the case and to warrant a good selection of the *simillimum*, we may note a reaction where a great number of symptoms appear after the administration of the remedy. If these are a return of former symptoms that have been forgotten, it is an indication that we are on the right road to recovery, and it is a truly homœopathic action. Old symptoms reappearing we know to be a step in the right direction, because we know the condition is being solved in the homœopathic manner, and by the law of the direction of cure : CURE TAKES PLACE FROM WITHIN OUTWARD, FROM ABOVE DOWNWARD, FROM THE IMPORTANT ORGANS TO THE LESS IMPORTANT ORGANS ; AND SYMPTOMS DISAPPEAR IN THE REVERSE ORDER OF THEIR APPEARANCE.

If, however, these are actually a number of new symptoms, it is an unfavourable sign. Old symptoms reappearing are a step in the right direction, as we know ; therefore a group of entirely new symptoms appearing after the administration of a remedy is evidence that we have made a decided step in the wrong direction. We have probably mixed the case.

We occasionally find another class of reactions after the administration of the remedy. In these cases, too, we find the appearance of new symptoms after the administration of the remedy, but in the first place these cases offered few symptoms for an adequate prescription. It is usually possible to get a complete symptomatic picture of the case if we take the necessary amount of care in taking the case, but we do occasionally meet cases where there is little presented in the way of symptoms, or the symptoms presented have little in the way of modifications as to modalities and concomitants upon which to base a satisfactory analysis of the case. Hahnemann deals with such cases in the *Organon*, Paragraphs 172-82. In these conditions where even the most careful case-taking fails to reveal an adequate basis for prescription of the *simillimum*, we may yet find that if the few symptoms are sufficiently well marked a remedy may be selected which will either eliminate the marked symptoms found in the first consideration of the case, with consequent general improvement, or there will be a development of more symptoms.

If there has been a general improvement, the first remedy was homœopathic to the case, and not alone to the few symptoms presented on our first consideration. In the second instance, the first remedy was probably one of a group of similars, and it has served to bring to light the other formerly hidden symptoms which were a definite part of the case. It has unfolded the case to us. In this instance, then, the closely related remedies to the one first administered will probably contain among them the *simillimum* which will be the remedy to cover and assist most in curing the complete case.

Even in these observations we must be very careful to consider whether we have administered a similar remedy that has unfolded the case to us, or whether our selection has been so far from the similar that we have merely mixed the case.

Diseased states are progressive, ever developing deeper and deeper manifestations. Disease is destruction ; cure is constructive development. Cure is always centrifugal, as growth is always centrifugal.

By careful observation of the symptoms before selecting the remedy and by careful observation of the reactions after the administration of the remedy, we may have the assurance that comes from intelligent comprehension of our work, and we can know when we are making satisfactory progress in each individual case.

What is the most necessary attribute of the homœopathic
  physician ? (*Answer :* His sense of perception.)
What are we to expect after the administration of the
  remedy ?
What are the most common reactions ? (*Answer :* <
  and > .)
What do we infer when the patient feels better, but the
  symptoms are < ?
What do we infer when the patient is weaker, but the
  symptoms are > ?
When there is actual aggravation of the diseased state, after
  the administration of the *simillimum*, what is our
  prognosis ?
Does the homœopathic remedy ever produce a fatal aggravation, if there has been no such indication present before ?
When actual aggravation of a diseased state gives a prognosis
  of a deep-acting disease after a deep-acting remedy has
  been administered what can we do to help the patient ?
  (*Answer :* Sometimes a complementary remedy, of less
  depth of action, will actually assist the patient to a place
  where cure may be carried out by the deep-acting
  simillimum ; or it would surely palliate the dangerous
  and distressing symptoms if no cure were possible.)
What is the sure guide for our prognosis ?
What is the most desirable reaction after administration of
  the remedy ? (*Answer :* A short, quick, strong aggravation, with closely following amelioration and recession
  of the symptoms in the order of cure.)
What do we infer when we find first a strong amelioration,
  then < ?
In cases seemingly proceeding to a perfect cure, when
  amelioration comes suddenly to a halt, what is our next
  step ? (*Answer :* Find out if the patient is doing
  something to interfere with the action of the remedy, or
  if it is just a cycle of the disease symptoms.)
What is the difference between an aggravation occurring
  immediately after the administration of the remedy, and
  one occurring two or three days after its administration ?
If we find too short an amelioration after administration of
  the remedy in chronic disease, what is our prognosis ?

What do we infer from the patient who seems to prove any remedy that may be given him ?

If many symptoms appear after the administration of the remedy, what must we consider ?

How do you know that the remedy has acted ? What is the first indication of it ?

What is the prognosis of the aggravation of the symptoms ?

What is the prognosis of the amelioration of the symptoms but the patient does not feel as well ?

Can you always depend upon what the patient says ?

In case of aggravation, and the patient is actually growing weaker, what does this indicate ?

When the patient feels better, but is growing weaker, what does this indicate ? (*Answer :* Reversal of the order of cure, symptoms are taking on a deeper form, although there may be actual amelioration of the more noticeable symptoms.)

Why do we have to observe closely the natural course of cure, after the remedy has been administered ?

Does this take precedence over what the patient tells us of the opinion he holds as to his improvement or less in condition ? Why ?

Chapter XV

DRUG PROVING

DRUGS have been used as the usual method of cure for disease since antiquity, and their derivations varied from simple herbs and substances to fearsome combinations from all imaginable sources. The preparation and administration of medicines was kept as a mystery for centuries, and the medicine man was held as superior and revered as a little more than mortal for his powers. Various doctrines of healing sprang up through the years ; perhaps the most interesting of these was the doctrine of signatures, founded on the belief that each member of the vegetable kingdom carried within itself the likeness of some organ or part of the human economy, as a sign that this particular plant was applicable to disturbances of that organ. That was probably the most consistent method among all the very ancient systems of applying drugs.

As medical knowledge progressed, occasional writers caught glimpses of better methods of drug application, but such light was rare and medical practice soon lapsed once more into the gloom of superstition. Paracelsus gained considerable insight into the action of drugs, and Halle, the Swedish physician, was a forerunner of Hahnemann in his deliberate experiments to discover the nature of certain remedies. These attempts were not co-ordinated, and made little impression upon the medical world. It was not until Hahnemann demanded to know the action of drugs upon the human organism that the work was taken up in an orderly way ; this demand, however, was not forthcoming until after he discovered the law of cure. The discovery of the law made it mandatory to know the action of drugs, and Hahnemann set to work to obtain that knowledge and called the work drug proving.

What is a drug ? And what do we do to prove a drug ?
In order to answer the question, What is a drug ? we

must go back and ask, What is life ? Continued action of those forces, through and upon the organs of the body, which preserve it from decay, this is life ; and health is that balanced action of these forces which preserves the integrity of all the parts. In this balance lies the conservation of the whole ; without this balance more or less destruction of the parts is the result, and the value of this balance is determined by the importance and number of organs or functions involved.

A drug is any material agent, in however attenuated form, the ingestion of which is capable of so disturbing this balance of the vital forces that the functioning of one or more organs of the body is no longer carried out to the best of the whole ; and any material substance capable of so acting on the living organism is a drug. Hence drugs are essentially destructive ; therein lies the difference between drugs and foods—drugs are destructive while foods are constructive. Both drugs and foods act upon the vital force which rules in all animate beings.

To ascertain the knowledge of a drug is to discover what disturbance of this balance it is capable of producing and what organs are affected ; how and what functional changes are made manifest. When we have discovered all this about a drug we can say we have a proving.

In order to be sure of the integrity of our work, we must demand three essential things :

(1) The quality of the drug must be pure ; it must be free from all mixture with other drugs, and it must possess all its active properties.

(2) The prover must possess the proper balance in functions and be in a normal, healthy state, so that we can estimate and weigh the amount of the disturbance caused when we deliberately upset the balance of health.

(3) The circumstances surrounding the prover must be those of his normal surroundings, so that the drug can express its action under conditions and circumstances normal to the prover, that any deviation from normal in the prover's condition cannot be attributed to different circumstances and conditions of his life, but directly to the action of the drug.

These three points must be maintained most carefully. The ordinary habits of life must be observed, and his ordinary work maintained ; otherwise changes from his routine might cause some deviation from his normal balance which would be attributed to the drug action.

All people do not make equally good provers. Some types are more susceptible to certain drug groups than are other types, and those who manifest susceptibility to the action of a drug to the point of developing symptoms must be secured for a satisfactory proving. Those who are peculiarly susceptible to a drug make the best provers, for it is the peculiarly susceptible who develop in the proving the peculiar, rare and characteristic symptoms of the drug ; yet those who are less susceptible cannot be rejected as provers provided they develop symptoms even in a small degree, as these serve to verify the symptoms produced in the extremely susceptible, and thus establish them as true symptoms and not chance observations. Not all provers will develop or give the identical symptomatology, some recording a complete symptom while others will record but a partial symptom.

In a consideration of food and the susceptible prover, in some instances an individual will manifest an idiosyncrasy to a certain food or group of foods. To this susceptible, the food becomes a drug, and the individual having this idiosyncrasy is merely manifesting his susceptibility to the possible drug properties in this food substance ; he will be the best possible prover of this drug.

The prover must be intelligent enough properly to appreciate and record the subjective symptoms as deviations from his normal conditions of life, as these subjective symptoms are of the utmost value. There is a vast difference in people in their ability both to perceive and to describe their subjective symptoms, therefore we must have a prover who has the gift of perception. We find the lack of perception in many patients who cannot describe their symptoms ; such people do not make good provers.

Honesty is a prerequisite of a good prover, for he must be very careful to record all phenomena as fact. Remember, a proving is a record of facts—facts that can be produced repeatedly in others ; therefore facts must be carefully recorded from the very beginning of the experiment ; yet we must avoid equally scepticism, imaginary phenomena or the over-colouring of the real ,facts. Remember always to treat a fact as a fact and do not try to add to or subtract from its importance ; it is not for the prover to sift the symptoms produced. Treat the facts as they are ; unless one can do this, he will not make a valuable prover.

At the beginning of this work, the prover must be in that state of mental, moral and physical equilibrium that is characteristic of a normal, healthy being. One who is subject to rapidly changing equilibrium on any one or all of these planes will not make a good prover.

Bear in mind the main and only object in conducting a proving : to discover the positive characteristics of the action of the drug on the vital energy of the human being ; to obtain a full knowledge of its action so that its powers can be readily distinguished from any other drug, *for the lawful application of the remedy in states of disturbed vital energy which we call disease.*

In making the record, all symptoms must be recorded, but we must not forget that many of these symptoms are held in common with many' other drugs ; while these symptoms possess a certain value in the final analysis, we must determine those symptoms of the greatest value, especially those which are the most peculiar and characteristic of the drug— the rare, unusual symptoms that distinguish it from all others, because these are the symptoms which will be the curative symptoms, in that they will be the guiding symptoms in selecting the remedy. The symptoms such as are held in common by many drugs are not of great value in the curative sphere. Every symptom must be recorded without bias or favour, otherwise we shall lose unwittingly some of the characteristic symptoms ; after all are recorded we can then compare all these symptoms with other drug provings.

So in making a proving two things are to be accomplished : a detailed record of the order of appearance of all symptoms, and an analysis of the symptoms. In making the analysis the three major points of all symptoms should be borne in mind : Location ; sensation ; and the modifying character of the symptoms, or modalities, together with the concomitant or apparently unrelated symptoms. The analysis is not complete until we have a comparison of the symptoms with those produced by other drug provings.

Having a clear view of the real objective of a proving, and having complied with all the requirements to produce such a proving, how do we proceed?

First, let us consider the dose. It may be we shall use the crude drug, or a low potency, or a high potency, depending upon the nature of the drug. How do we determine which to use? There are certain considerations which are sufficiently stable for guiding rules. From an apparently inert substance, such as *Lycopodium*, *Carbo veg.* or *Graphites*, we can obtain a good proving only from a high potency ; therefore we may take as an axiom : ANY DRUG WHICH IN ITS NATURAL STATE AFFECTS THE VITAL ENERGY BUT LITTLE WILL DEVELOP A PROVING ONLY IN A HIGH POTENCY. Other drugs having a very strong action upon the human economy in their natural state, such as *Lobelia*, *Ipecac.*, *Cicuta* or *Tavacum*, may be used in a crude form : ANY DRUG WHICH IN ITS NATURAL STATE DISTURBS THE VITAL ENERGY TO FUNCTIONAL MANIFESTATIONS ONLY MAY BE PROVEN IN A CRUDE FORM. Still other drugs, such as the *Mercurius* group, which are actively poisonous in the crude form, can be proven only in the high potencies : ANY DRUG WHICH IN ITS NATURAL STATE DISTURBS THE VITAL ENERGY TO DESTRUCTIVE MANIFESTATIONS SHOULD BE PROVEN ONLY IN A POTENTIATED FORM.

In other words, we determine the plane of the drug we wish to use by a consideration of the object we desire to attain. The object of the proving is to produce the characteristics of the drug as they are manifest in diseased states.

The comparatively inert substances will produce no symptoms ; at best a very few symptoms of low value in the crude state, and these are not characteristic of the drug ; either no symptoms are produced, or if perchance a few symptoms are produced they are not strikingly peculiar of the drug. The inert substances are expelled from the body before they reach the dynamis of the system, the vital energy.

In the provings of active or corrosive poisons in low or

crude state the same thing is true : they are valueless because the grosser irritating symptoms are the result of mechanical disturbances and the few strikingly characteristic symptoms of the drug are never observed. The corrosives are expelled very quickly in the crude state because of the violence of their action, and so do not influence the vital energy to produce characteristic symptoms ; therefore the symptoms that are produced are of little value because they are common to all corrosive poisons.

The susceptibility of the patient or prover must be taken into consideration ; this regulates and gives us direction as to the quantity of the drug to be taken. The greater the susceptibility, the less the quantity required to react upon the vital force, for if the organism is overwhelmed suddenly at first we may get only generic symptoms and so fail to obtain the characteristic symptoms and thus fail in our object. On the other hand, if he is only moderately susceptible, we may obtain valuable results from larger doses. Our standard should be TO USE THE DOSE AND QUANTITY THAT WILL THOROUGHLY PERMEATE THE ORGANISM AND MAKE ITS ESSENTIAL IMPRESS UPON THE VITAL FORCE AND THUS AFFECT THE FUNCTIONAL SPHERE OF HIS BODY. This is best accomplished when a gradual impress is made, rather than a sudden onslaught, for then we would bring into the picture alarm because of violent functional disturbances, which certainly defeats our object. So when the first dose is followed by no marked symptoms, a second dose may be given, and then a period of waiting until some symptoms appear. If after the interval of waiting there is no appearance of symptoms, another dose may be given. By this gradual introduction of the drug the system becomes pervaded by its action and tolerates it, and responds to its specific impression and we obtain its characteristics.

In carrying out the provings by the higher potencies only the very susceptible will respond ; this is no reflection upon the value of the provings made from the higher potencies, because we only obtain the characteristics of the remedy from such provings. The fact that the more obtuse prover does not respond does not have any weight, for under any potency proving he will only produce generic symptoms—

symptoms held in common with the whole family we are proving. This contributes nothing to the knowledge of the drug which will be of value in the cure of disease. Neither does the fact that the obtuse prover does not respond to develop a proving of the remedy influence the value of the drug in its application to the sick, for when the vital energy is disturbed, it is far more susceptible to influence from a drug than when the vital energy is in a state of equilibrium. From the very nature of the case, symptoms produced from the higher potencies are genuine and are of the highest value as a curative agent.

The repetition of the dose will be governed by the nature of the drug and the reaction of the vital energy. Some drugs, like *Silica* or *Lycopodium,* are slow in action and should be administered at long intervals, while others are quick to give a reaction and shorter in their duration. However, this is an absolutely dependable rule : NEVER REPEAT THE DOSE WHILE SYMPTOMS ARE MANIFEST FROM THE DOSE ALREADY TAKEN. This is the same rule applied to the proving as governs the administration of the remedy in the cure of sickness : NEVER REPEAT YOUR REMEDY SO LONG AS IT CONTINUES TO ACT. The reason is as obvious in one case as in the other. It is absolutely essential to obtain a proving of real value and integrity as showing forth the characteristics of the drug and the order of the symptoms in their development.

Symptoms are produced in sequences, and it is important to know the first effects as shown in the symptoms, the sequence of their appearance and their duration ; and a repetition of the dose defeats our purpose by upsetting this sequence, and continued repetition destroys the knowledge of the latest symptoms to appear, which are always the most valuable because they are the most characteristic, and farthest removed from possible pathogenetic action.

The duty of recording the symptoms in their order of appearance is very important, and quite as important is the duty of recording the concomitant symptoms, their associates, which, WHILE SEEMINGLY UNRELATED TO THE CASE, YET BEAR A CLOSE RELATIONSHIP IN THAT THEY APPEAR AT THE SAME TIME AND IN ASSOCIATION WITH THE OTHER SYMPTOMS.

The value of the symptom record is largely based upon the order of appearance of symptoms and their associated or concomitant symptoms. The farther removed the symptom appears from the dose the more important its value. Not all symptoms are of equal value, so that much valuable data is added to the proving by carefully observing the sequences.

The prover should be a faithful recorder of symptoms, not only their sequence, but he must be very explicit as to the character of all sensations : pain, dull, stinging, piercing, throbbing, etc. The exact locality of the sensations, such as pain, must be given ; if it is shooting, where it starts and the direction of its course ; if it is one-sided, in what direction does it move, or does it go to the other side ? If so, does it remain there or return to the first side ? Not the least important of the sensations are those which are difficult to describe directly, and can only be given by the introduction, " sensation as if . . . ". It is these which make the characteristic proving, and are identification marks of the remedy.

Remember, all symptoms have location, sensation, and the aggravations and ameliorations, plus their concomitants ; these should all be recorded faithfully in every proving. Too much care cannot be exercised in recording the direction of symptoms, the times of aggravation and amelioration, the effect of atmospheric changes, and positions taken by the patient in order to obtain relief. We must record the effects of position upon the patient, both for aggravation and amelioration ; the positions he takes in sleep ; what effects are produced from standing, walking, sitting, lying ; if changes are produced while lying on the right side, the left side, or back ; what effect motion or rest has upon his symptoms, and especially the changes of posture, such as rising up or lying down or from continued motion ; the particular kind of motion that affects him. How do eating and drinking affect him ? How does sleeping affect him ? How do these things affect him at the time, and afterward, and in relation to each other ? What is the condition produced by being in the presence of associates, or in crowds, or by being alone ? We must consider everything that tends to increase or diminish the patient's equilibrium.

Too much emphasis cannot be placed upon the faithful recording of these manifestations, because it is in these aggravations and ameliorations and attending circumstances that we find the characteristics that make the drug of value as a curative agent.

One is struck with the thoroughness of Hahnemann and the earlier provers, by the great amount of detail with which the records of those provings were made in comparison with many of the newer provings, and this is the reason why the older provings are of so much value. They produced the expression of the drug, the very living elements of the proving. All the facts were recorded ; and this we must remember in our own work of recording, that all facts must be recorded, for we are not to judge what is essential or what is insignificant ; we do not know when some apparently insignificant symptom may become of much value in the grand total of a complete symptomatology.

In making the record of many provings of the same drug there is an inclination to omit as insignificant a symptom recorded by only one prover, yet, like the 3 a.m. cough of *Kali carb.*, this one symptom may be of inestimable value in prescribing. Had this symptom not been recorded because it was considered insignificant, having appeared in but one record, how much would have been lost to the record of *Kali carb.* !

Objective symptoms play but a small part in the record, for they are of little value as curative symptoms. However, to be complete the record should embrace these symptoms.

The great essential to be required of the prover is to record all symptoms faithfully ; then the physician can give the proper value to the finished record, remembering always that the real and only object of a proving is to record a living personality whom we will be able to recognize when we meet in the sick room.

CHAPTER XVI

THE SECOND PRESCRIPTION

AFTER studying a chronic case and after deciding on the remedy, having given each symptom its proper evaluation, and having administered the *simillimum*, we expect some action, some response. After the patient shows the desired reaction, there may and probably will come a time when the physician is called upon to meet a symptom picture once more. This is the time when he must consider the second prescription.

Strictly speaking, the first prescription is the prescription that first reacts. A physician may make a mistake and not select a remedy that is similar, consequently with no reaction. Thus while we may seem to be looking for a second prescription, we are in reality looking for a first prescription to which the patient will react. In other words, the prescription must be considered as the *simillimum*. Unless the patient reacts to the administration of a remedy and it has produced an effect, it is not a true prescription, for it is quite evident that it is not the *simillimum*. It is really bungling.

The second prescription may be a repetition of the first. On the other hand, the reaction may have been such that an antidote is required ; or the first remedy having taken care of a part of the symptoms, a complement of the first prescription may be demanded. In order to meet the situation intelligently, after the remedy has reacted, the case must be thoroughly restudied.

In general, if the first prescription has had a beneficial reaction, that remedy should be allowed to complete its work to the fullest extent. In such conditions, the second prescription would be a repetition of the first ; and since a remedy should not be changed without very good reasons, it is probable that the remedy may be repeated at the necessary intervals through a whole range of potencies, securing the full amount of good from each potency before passing on to the next.

The reaction to the correct prescription is that the striking features, the peculiar features, the concomitant symptoms on which the choice of the remedy was based, are the first symptoms to be removed ; thus the guiding symptoms of the case have been obliterated. The picture has been almost erased, and only the trivial symptoms are left. Now if the remedy is repeated at this stage, the cycle of cure is broken ; for the guiding symptoms will surely return only when the action of the remedy is exhausted. If there is no interference with the action of the remedy, the indications which give us the clue to our next step will present themselves. One of the hardest things for a physician to do is to keep his hands off at this stage. If the remedy is administered at this stage we will find an intermingling of drug symptoms, so that no intelligent prescription can be made.

If the first prescription has not acted curatively, or it has not been permitted to act to its fullest extent, it is impossible to get second observations ; but suppose that the first prescription was correct, and that it has been given plenty of time to act without interference :—

If the case has come to a standstill or if the first prescription has caused changes in the symptomatology that remain, that do not vary greatly for some little time, it is time to go over the case again with the second prescription in mind. While these changes are going on, no orderly symptoms can be gathered and no rational observations made. If we have given time for the proper reaction and the fuller development of the case, having allowed the natural period of rest, the time has come to make a minute observation upon the return of the original symptoms, which should be our first consideration.

They may not return as strong or marked as they appeared before the first prescription, but we must look carefully for the return of the original symptoms. It is while the action of the remedy is going on that the vital principle is re-established in the economy ; and while this process is going on we will not find the return of the original symptoms. The length of time varies in different individuals

10

and in different remedies ; it may be a few weeks and it may be months.

Now what are we to do at this time ? Without symptoms we cannot prescribe intelligently. Symptoms are the only guide to the remedy. The duty of the physician is plainly marked : to await the return of the symptom picture. In chronic conditions we may be quite sure that the symptoms will return, for it is very rarely that we can cure a case with one prescription. When the symptoms return, they may be changed as to their intensity ; sometimes they return in a less intense form and sometimes they are increased in intensity. The fact that the original symptoms return is a very good omen. It shows that the first prescription was correct. In this case there is very little that we need in the way of information beyond this, because we know that the remedy was right and the patient can be cured. In this case the remedy must be a repetition of the first prescription.

Another class of cases we must consider are those that present a number of new symptoms which appear to take the place of the old symptoms. The old symptoms do not return, but are replaced by an entirely different symptom group. In these conditions we must restudy the case entirely in the pathogenesis of the remedy we have already given, and find if the new symptoms that have appeared are in the pathogenesis of the remedy. If this is so, we may find that this condition comes from a partial proving of the remedy, or we may find that these appear from a different cause. This is an important point. We must determine from the patient whether he has ever had any of these symptoms before in any former sicknesses or under any other conditions. We must go over these points carefully to see if we cannot elicit from the patient the history of these symptoms. Sometimes we get these relationships from the patient and sometimes from the family.

If these are old symptoms, we not only chose our first prescription correctly but it has eliminated the newest symptoms and uncovered an older layer, in the proper order of cure ; but if we can get no history of the patient having had these symptoms before, and if they are not in the pathogenesis of the remedy, we have made a mistake in the first prescription, and it has changed the direction of the disease. Here, if it is possible, we must antidote the remedy.

After having given the antidotal remedy and a little time for the patient to rest, we should study the case again from the beginning ; and the second remedy should correspond more particularly to the new symptoms than to the old, but both the present symptoms and the former symptoms must be considered. If we do our work carefully, this second prescription will cause the new symptoms to disappear and it will probably remove the old symptoms as well.

We may have to repeat the process several times before we really overcome the difficulty, but each time that it is done makes the next step more difficult and we must proceed with increasing caution after having made the mistake.

After the first prescription has been made sometimes the patient will come to a standstill. The symptoms have changed in an orderly way ; new symptoms have come up ; but finally the symptoms have all retired in the reverse order to a former state and are hardly of sufficient importance to be considered. The patient will acknowledge that the troublesome symptoms have disappeared, and that he has little in the way of symptoms to report, but he does not feel well ; there is no general sense of well-being, yet he can scarcely tell you why and where he does not feel well.

In such states we should wait until we are quite sure the remedy has ceased to act. There are remedies that have a " do nothing " stage in their unfolding, and we must be sure, before repeating the remedy, that the first prescription has entirely run out its cycle. If we have found a " do nothing " stage, it may be but a part of the remedy cycle ; if so, the remedy is still acting and to repeat the remedy at this time could do no good and might do harm. In other words, this " do nothing " stage is an expression of the pathogenesis of the remedy as manifesting itself in the curative process, and by a little more patient waiting the patient will be ready for the next prescription. In these " do nothing " states no other remedy can fill in, because there are no strong indications for another remedy and the symptomatology has not altered to any marked degree except by lessening in intensity, and since there has been little change and no marked new symptoms have arisen, we have no guides for another remedy.

Then we must consider when to change the remedy for the second prescription. Besides the condition we have already spoken of, where new symptoms have appeared and there is an entire change, if the marked symptoms have disappeared and a new group of symptoms have appeared, with no relation to the former history of the patient, a new remedy must be considered.

Suppose in a chronic case these constitutional symptoms have been correctly met, and have gone through a range of potencies from the lowest up to the highest, and that they have all acted curatively, and the case has come to a stand-still. After repeating the remedy we get no reaction. This constitutional remedy should be allowed to continue its curative action as long as it can be maintained and even if the symptoms have changed somewhat do not change the remedy as long as the patient shows improvement ; but on the other hand, if the patient is not improving and there has been a change in the symptoms we can safely retake the case for the consideration of another remedy. We must make sure, however, that these symptoms are different from those the patient felt earlier, or have not been covered up by later developments, for a patient tends to become accustomed to certain symptoms and almost forgets that he has had them. If asked about them, he often replies that " they are nothing ; he has always had them ", but these may be an important part of the symptomatology and we may elicit the fact that these are just a return of old symptoms that have not been previously noticed or reported. On the other hand, it may be that we have really had all the action we can expect from the remedy that has been administered, and it is time to consider another remedy, since the first one has carried the patient as far as possible. A safe rule for procedure is : WHEN IN DOUBT, WAIT. In other words, never leave a constitutional remedy, that has proven the *simillimum* for a considerable period, until you have extracted from it all the benefit that the remedy can contribute. Then, and only then, are you justified in changing the remedy.

It is quite possible that in making a second prescription

we may find the *simillimum* to be complementary to the first. This is particularly well illustrated in the sicknesses of child life. There are often repeated tendencies for colds. The patient seems to be getting colds all the while, and a remedy like *Belladonna* may seem to be indicated and will cure the acute condition promptly. We may do this two or three times before we realize that these recurrences are an acute exacerbation of a chronic condition, and while *Belladonna* acts promptly and effectively, it is only because it is a complementary remedy to the underlying chronic *Calcarea* state. *Pulsatilla* may be as effective in acute manifestations while the constitutional condition calls for *Silica*. It is so with many remedies.

Then we may find constitutional conditions that require, for a complete cure, a succession of remedies, one remedy following another to good advantage. This may be a process of zigzagging a case to a cure because of lack of knowledge of our remedies or because the case does not unfold before us when we first consider it.

There is another possible reason for the successful succession of remedies. The first prescription may remove all the symptoms of one miasmatic condition, when suddenly a condition will arise which shows a basic condition of one of the other miasms. One miasm may have been submerged under another, and after the first has been removed by the *simillimum*, the second shows, and the plan of attack must be changed to include as weapons another group of stigmatic remedies. We cannot expect to eradicate any stigma with a single dose of any remedy, but we may so improve the manifestations that the underlying condition may show itself, perhaps later to return to the first miasm again.

In these chronic conditions, no prescription, either first or second, can be made without careful, thorough study of the case and the sequence of symptoms. It is only by working out the case with the repertories that we are able to see clearly the indicated constitutional remedy in the light of the symptoms that have been cured or relieved. It is only then that we can administer another remedy intelligently and with confidence.

CHAPTER XVII

SUSCEPTIBILITY

EVERYTHING that has life is more or less influenced by circumstances and environment. This is true in the natural growth and development of the vegetable kingdom. Certain flora develop fully only in certain altitudes and when swept by the constant moisture of the ocean ; they will take on an entirely different form under other circumstances and environment. The trees in the open show the constant effect of pressure from prevailing winds. Years ago Connecticut horticulturists raised quantities of peaches ; then suddenly all the peach trees died, and for about fifty years no peaches were grown in the state. Then Mr. J. H. Hale discovered that peaches throve only in soil rich in potash. Returning to Connecticut, he analysed the soil where peaches had failed, and found there was very little or no potash in that soil. If potash is supplied, luscious peaches will grow abundantly.

The same susceptibility to influences is true in the animal kingdom. Animals from certain parts of the earth's surface develop peculiarities of their own which are entirely different from their close relatives elsewhere. They can withstand certain influences and hold their own under adverse conditions which would be fatal to another of the same species developed under differing circumstances. In other words, they develop a protective immunity against their environmental conditions. The polar bear is immune to the rigours of the Arctic, but is susceptible and soon succumbs to the influence of warm climates. The Bengal tiger thrives in the humidity of the Indian jungles ; other members of the tiger family have adapted themselves to the altitude and rarefied atmosphere of the slopes of the Himalayas and the searching winds of those heights ; either is susceptible to the ravages incident to a change of temperature.

We may define susceptibility primarily as the reaction of the organism to external and internal influences. While we may point out striking illustrations of susceptibility in the vegetable kingdom or among the lower animals, the best illustrations are to be found among those human beings with whom we come in contact. We see very frequently the susceptibility to climatic conditions, as well as all other phases of environment. One person will thrive in a rigorous climate where another will become seriously ill; one will thrive in dampness to which another would succumb. Altitude affects some individuals kindly and some adversely. The seashore improves one man's condition while it makes another man ill.

The power of assimilation and nutrition is one of the phases of susceptibility. One easily assimilates a certain kind of food while another finds the same food indigestible. " One man's meat is another man's poison."

Human beings are susceptible to infection and contagion in varying degrees. One man will become infected in contact with diseased individuals while another will experience no ill effects whatever. One person is made ill by noxious plants while another man can handle them with impunity. Certain people are capable of making a wonderful proving of a drug, whereas others will show no reaction whatever.

All these reactions have to do with susceptibility

In analysing susceptibility, we find it is very largely an expression of a vacuum in the individual. This is illustrated by the desire for food. The vacuum attracts and pulls for the things most needed, that are on the same plane of vibration as the want in the body.

Contagious diseases thrive in childhood because of the extreme susceptibility of the miasmatic influence; this susceptibility has an attractive force which draws to itself the disease which is on the same plane of vibration and which tends to correct this miasmatic deficiency. After having drawn to itself this other disease manifestation, the child becomes immune to further onslaughts of the same condition ; his system has become somewhat cleared by this attraction of what Hahnemann calls a " similar disease " condition.

Susceptibility varies in degree in different patients, and at different times in the same patient. Homœopathic application of a remedy is an illustration of meeting the susceptibility and filling the vacuum that is present in the sick individual. In other words, the vibrations of the sick individual call aloud for something to meet the need. The proving of the remedy on a healthy individual gives us the basis of similarity of remedies to sick individuals because in a proving the remedy produces an artificial susceptibility similar to the susceptibility of the sick individual. The application of the homœopathic remedy in sickness satisfies this natural susceptibility. No matter how little reaction of the remedy develops in the proving on a healthy individual, the susceptibility is greatly accentuated in sickness. The indications for a remedy show the susceptibility in a marked degree and the patient will respond, because the similar potentized remedy is always stronger than the susceptibility so that it fully satisfies the morbid condition. This satisfaction is based on a universal law governing the symptomatically similar remedy. A patient may be susceptible to a number of remedies, but the greatest susceptibility is manifest in the most similar; in other words, the *simillimum*. They would be influenced somewhat, however, by the nearly similar.

Susceptibility can be increased, diminished or destroyed. It therefore becomes a state of lowered resistance or attraction.

Dr. J. J. Garth Wilkinson, in *Epidemic Man and His Visitations*, says :

One man catches scarlet fever from another man, but catches it because he is *vis minor* to the disease, which to him alone is *vis major*. His neighbour does not catch it ; his strength passes it by as no concern of his. It is the first man's foible that is the prime reason of his taking the complaint. He is a vacuum for its pressure. The cause why he succumbed was in him long before the infector appeared. Susceptibility to a disease is sure in the individual or his race to be (come) that disease in time. . . . Susceptibility in organism, mental or bodily, is equivalent to *state*. State involves the attitude of organizations to internal causes and to external circumstances. It is all the resource of defence or the way of yielding. The taking on of states is the history of human life. . . . In health we live and act and resist without knowing it. In disease we live but suffer ; and know *ourself* in conscious or unconscious exaggeration.

It is incumbent upon us to recognize, conserve and utilize normal susceptibility, to physical environments, to foods, to remedies and to toxic agencies. It should be our aim never to use any agent or anything of any nature, or to adopt any procedure, that would in the least diminish or destroy this power of susceptibility and the reaction of the organism in its normal manner. Upon this normal susceptibility and reaction depends the status of health. To do anything to diminish or destroy the normal reaction is not the province of a physician ; rather it is the province of the physician to conserve natural susceptibility, for without a recognition of this power all our efforts as physicians would be worthless. It is just as much the province of the physician to exercise conservation of susceptibility in the organism that it may act defensively against a toxin, contagion or infection, as it is to have this susceptibility react constructively to food and drink or to the curative remedy. Again, it is just as natural and important for the organism to react pathogenetically to the size and power of a dose of poison as it is for it to react to the demand for food.

We must lay particular stress on demanding the conservation of normal susceptibility in the care of the sick, for in sickness susceptibility is exaggerated and we must be very careful to do nothing to impair it, for it is through this exaggerated reaction that we find our clue to the similar remedy. In sickness it is essential to remember that it is only in the administration of the similar remedy that susceptibility is satisfied. All our efforts must be gauged by this one question : *Does the remedy satisfy the demands of this exaggerated susceptibility ?*

We cannot stress too much the necessity of adhering strictly to the law of similars in meeting these susceptibilities. Many medicines or preparations are introduced into the organism either by mouth or by injection into the blood stream, that have no basis of similarity to the susceptibility of the patient, and which are therefore destructive to the restoration of normal susceptibility. When such procedures are adopted on any other basis than symptom similarity, the esults are either palliative or suppressive, and the ultimate result is that the patient is worse than before, or complete destruction takes place.

Professor James Ewing, of Cornell University Medical College, is quoted by Dr. Stuart Close as making the following statements in 1909 in a lecture upon *Immunity* :

The effort to produce passive immunity against the various infections by means of sera may fail in spite of the destruction of all the bacteria present in the body, by reason of the endotoxins thrown out in the process of bacteriolysis resulting from the serum injections.

The action of endotoxins of all kinds is similar : there is a reduction of temperature but an active degeneration of the organs—a *status infectiosus*. Thus sterile death is produced where cultures from the organs and tissues show that the bacteria in question have all been destroyed ; *but the animal dies*.

This problem of the endotoxins is at present the stone wall of serum therapy.   .   .   .

An animal whose serum is normally bacteriolytic may, on immunization, lose this power ; the bacteria living in the serum, but not producing symptoms. Thus, a rabbit's serum is normally bacteriolytic to the typhoid bacillus, but the rabbit is susceptible to infection. If, however, the rabbit is highly immunized the serum is no longer bactericidal, the typhoid bacilli living in the serum, but the animal not being susceptible of infection. The animal dies.

It seems therefore that the effort must be made in the future to enable the tissue and the bacteria to live together in peace rather than to produce a state where the serum is destructive to the bacteria.

In Professor Ewing's illustration he shows the destruction or impairment of susceptibility of the organism to react to the stimulus of either sera or bacilli. Total destruction of the reactivity of the body means death. Partial destruction or serious impairment may render the patient a chronic invalid with impossibility of cure. With the destruction of the reactivity the corresponding destruction of the bacilli is not accomplished and the patient is in a deplorable condition of chronic invalidism.

Another attempt to forcibly regulate body reaction is through the use of antiseptics, which is another means of destroying bacilli, but which at the same time destroys normal susceptibility. The *Boston Surgical Journal* has shown that antiseptics used in cases of tonsillitis increase the inflammation, prolong the disease and retard convalescence. It is demonstrated that in the effort to diminish bacteria in the crypts, which generate toxins, the period required for the formation of the requisite amount of antibodies was unduly prolonged. In other words, it was demonstrated that living organisms, even if diseased, have some means of self-protection ; and that, other things being equal, the automatic formation of antitoxins or antibodies goes on at about an equal pace with the generation of toxins. However, in the use of antiseptics other things are not equal, and it is impossible for the body to exert its normal powers of self defence, since its normal susceptibility is lowered. This destructive action of antiseptics on the living cells and phagocytic leucocytes of the patient was also pointed out in the *Boston Surgical Journal*, as contra-indicating their use. In destroying these bodies we are destroying the physical basis of life itself, since antiseptics powerful enough to destroy cells of one type must certainly have an equally destructive effect on other cells. The investigation further demonstrated that the depression of the vitality thus caused resulted in fever and cervical adenitis due to an increased absorption of the toxins. Increase of fever is a manifestation of the vital reaction and resistance toward disease on the part of the organism ; this normal reactivity shows an increase in leucocytes and an increased production also of antibodies and antitoxins. This normal process should never be interfered with, because it represents the normal reaction and resistance of the vital energy, and it is Nature's method of protecting the organism.

The human economy has inherited many tendencies from the accumulations of its ancestral heritage. These tendencies show themselves in child life in the great number of so-called children's diseases, which are nothing more nor less than an inward turmoil of bringing to the surface and expelling certain conditions ; again, these eruptions are a lack of ability on the part of the patient to create a similar state within his own economy to satisfy the susceptibility. In other words, by the lack of the applied similar remedy, the susceptibility is not met ; therefore Nature steps in with the laws of susceptibility and an influence is attracted which blooms forth as an infectious or contagious disease, so as to most fully satisfy this susceptibility. When the susceptibility of this particular state has once been satisfied by an expression of the similar condition, a partial cure has taken place and they can no more develop the reaction to a similar infection.

This tendency of human economies is brought out still further by the susceptibilities of whole families toward certain types of diseases. This is often seen when whole families succumb to certain types of diseases that leave their neighbours untouched. This again is governed by the law of susceptibility, which attracts unto itself and has particular affinity for certain diseased conditions because they are similar to the constitutional condition. Just as certain traits of susceptibility are manifest in family groups, so we find the tendency predominates in certain racial groups one race being particularly susceptible to certain diseases which touch another race but lightly. It is because the similar condition has remained unsupplied through generations, and the laws of attraction and susceptibility are manifesting their powers.

Thus we see that susceptibility and reaction are basic principles, and are very closely allied to the problems of immunization. A proper concept of these principles is something that the homœopathic physician must seriously consider ; the interplay of these principles must become as second nature to him, if he wishes to use well the forces of nature in healing the sick. THE SIMILAR REMEDY, OR THE SIMILAR DISEASE, SATISFIES SUSCEPTIBILITY AND ESTABLISHES IMMUNITY.

CHAPTER XVIII

SUPPRESSION

In the dissertations on the vital energy we pointed out that it was this force which was the expression of life itself, and through its power of development and control in itself and by itself it maintains the harmonious working, the state of equilibrium, which is perfect health. There are external forces which may have an impress upon vital energy, yet that allow it to work in undisturbed harmony ; and there are external forces that have great influence in inhibiting its normal functioning. When the normal function is inhibited the immediate reaction is a lack of harmony and a warped and suppressed functioning of the vital force, so that disease conditions are produced with the attendant symptoms and irregular functions of the body.

Let us consider some of these external features that may thus suppress the normal functions of the vital force, and through the vital force the normal functioning of the body. Such conditions as shell-shock, fright, fear, excessive joy, intense unsatisfied longing for mate or offspring, unrequited love, grief from loss of family or friends, business apprehensions and worries, disappointed ambitions, extreme fatigue or exhaustion ; all these forces have an influence upon the vital energy, and so warp and suppress its natural functioning that a train of symptoms is produced, varying in their manifestations, but each varying widely from the natural expressions of the vital energy. We often see cases where these suppressing emotions not only affect profoundly the single individual, but extend their influence to the next generation through the effect on a nursing mother.

The palliative effect of medicines in physiological form is a condition that we see over and over again, and we can observe the sequence of suppressive action, the results being first palliation and then suppression or an actual aggravation of the first condition. There are always the primary and secondary actions as a result of physiological dosage, and we see it well expressed in Paragraph 59 of the *Organon*, where Hahnemann says :

Such palliative antipathic remedies were never employed in allaying the prominent symptoms of protracted diseases, without being followed in a few hours by the contrary condition, i.e. the return of the evil, often seriously aggravated.

The paragraph continues, speaking of the use of opium in suppressing coughs, and the use of the same drug in diarrhœa, and coffee producing exhilaration, and other physiological primary effects in common practice ; then he goes on to show the secondary effects as being but an aggravation of the first condition, or an entirely different group of symptoms of deeper significance.

The homœopathic physician constantly comes across drug effects in physiological form which have suppressed the natural expression of disease. The one thing we should always bear in mind and should hold as our aim is to allow the vital force to express itself in its own chosen way when it is deranged. It is only when it shows itself clearly and without interruption in its natural development that we get a clear picture of the diseased state, and the administration of physiological medicine at such times changes the whole picture, suppressing one symptom after another until there is no expression of the true condition of the patient.

The immediate effect of this method of treatment is a suppression but if persisted in and continued over a period of time it has the effect of driving the vital energy to express itself in some other form, and usually in a deeper and more vital organ.

As an illustration, consider the use of opium and its derivatives for the suppression of coughs. If this treatment is continued for any length of time, instead of a cough we find the patient has become subject to a condition far more serious, for he has developed a chronic state of night cough ; each time it is suppressed it is driven still deeper, and the patient soon develops fever, night sweats, and a general hectic condition. This may happen in simple coughs. It may happen in pneumonic coughs. The danger of this suppression is very great, as can easily be noticed, especially in pneumonias, where the least suppression is often fatal.

Likewise in diarrhœas, the suppression of a diarrhœa will often produce constipation, then fever and a tendency to delirium. One who remembers the time when cholera infantum was so prevalent will remember also that many children who had received opium to stop the diarrhœa (which it promptly did) developed the next day a hydrocephaloid state and succumbed to the ravages of opium rather than to the ravages of the disease. The present indiscriminate use of the salicylates and coal tar derivatives in rheumatic and allied states invariably sends the trouble to the central organs, especially to the heart.

The present-day advertising of proprietary articles for the relief of pain, such as aspirin, and the consequent indiscriminate use of such preparations is exceedingly harmful, for it suppresses once more the danger signal of pain, and it always covers the condition but never removes it, rendering it possible to appear in a much exaggerated and more dangerous manifestation in some other organ, or in a much more serious condition in the same organ.

Another form of suppression that is very frequently seen is the external application of drug preparations for the removal of skin manifestations, such as eczema. These skin manifestations can be removed by the external use of drug preparations. This, however, does not cure the diseased condition, and the chronic miasm that has been expressed through the skin manifestations is forced to hide its head, but it surely will still be present in the organism and express itself in some deeper and more vital part, nearer the centre of vitality. If this course of treatment is persistently continued and the condition continually suppressed, the patient becomes nearly impossible of cure. The danger from these suppressions is very great, for the longer they are suppressed the more likely they are to take on nervous and mental manifestations, striking at the very seat of life and reason, and there expressing itself.

Hahnemann's *Organon*, Paragraph 61, gives us the following :

Had physicians correctly observed and considered the deplorable results of the antipathic application of medicines, they would long ago have discovered the great truth, that the true method of performing permanent cures must be the exact counterpart of such antipathic treatment.

They would have perceived that, whenever the opposite or antipathic administration of medicine produced a brief period of alleviation, this would subside, only to be followed by one of aggravation, and that, consequently, the process should have been reversed; that is to say, the homœopathic application of medicines according to their symptom-similitude would have brought about a lasting and perfect cure, provided that, instead of large quantities of medicine, the most minute doses had been employed. Notwithstanding the experience of many centuries, physicians did not recognize this great and salutary truth, they appear to have ignored entirely the results of treatment above described, as well as the other fact, that no physician ever effected a permanent cure of an inveterate disease, unless some drug of predominant homœopathic effect had been by chance embodied in his prescription nor were they able to comprehend that every rapid and perfect cure, accomplished by nature without the aid of human skill, was always produced by a similar disease coming to the one already present.

Another source of suppression is the attempt to suppress the natural secretions of the body, like the perspiration in the armpits and the perspiration of the feet, by the use of medicinal powders. This forbids the elimination of waste matter through the natural channels and this waste must be taken up in other parts of the body and the attempt made to eliminate them through these other channels. In this way much harm may be done, and while the local suppressions may be entirely successful, the constitutional manifestations are inimical to health.

Under the suppression of secretions we often find the suppression of the menses by cold baths, or the sudden suppression of sweat by plunging in for a cooling swim after exertion or in hot weather. Here, too, we find the resulting action on the vital force, with the disturbance taking on grave, or even dangerous, forms.

A frequent form of suppression in modern days is the removal of disturbing organs by surgical means, again forbidding the expression of the vital force through its chosen organs, where it has expressed itself in a diseased state of the tonsils, the teeth, the sinuses, or any other part of the economy. The particular disturbance is shown by the symptom picture of the patient. In removing the tonsils, the teeth, or other organs by surgical operation we are dealing with the end-product and not with the vital energy. We are cutting off the manifestation of disease and are doing nothing to set in order the vital energy or to prevent further disease manifestations. These diseased conditions have developed as an expression of the inward turmoil and distress under which the whole individual suffers.

These are but a few of the common suppressions caused by either physicians or laymen, or from circumstances, and but a few of the forms that are constantly met. It is the privilege of the homœopathic physician to relieve these distressed conditions and to set the vital energy in order, thus enabling it to function properly.

No greater crime can be committed against the human economy than to aid and abet these suppressions, for these may be the direct cause of many constitutional diseases, and the symptoms are in their natural state always the expression of constitutional conditions. Suppression is the source of many functional disturbances.

The homœopathic physician is the only physician who is equipped to deal with these conditions, for his province and the fundamental principle of his work is the proper co-ordination and normal functioning of the body, the mind and the spirit ; and it is only when the three spheres of man co-ordinate to develop in their normal way that harmony and health can be maintained and preserved.

Chapter XIX

THE LAW OF PALLIATION

Physicians who have been somewhat trained along homœopathic lines manifest more confusion in the treatment of incurable diseases than in almost any other field of medicine. When faced with incurable cases, the thought occurs to a great many physicians to administer palliative measures in an effort to alleviate suffering and to attempt to hide from the patient and from the family the real seriousness of the situation. Although they may mean well, it is an effort expended in the wrong direction, and does more harm than can well be estimated. There is no place in the field of medicine where obliteration of symptoms will cause so much confusion, so there is no possibility of accurate prescribing, as in these incurable cases.

The basis of cure is the fundamental law of similars. The law of similars is the fundamental law also in the palliation of incurable states. The administration of narcotics and sedatives suppresses symptoms and destroys the power of elimination by locking up the secretions in all states so completely that we cannot get a true picture of the condition of the vital force and energy upon which we must evaluate our symptomatology. The result of palliative treatment by the use of narcotics demands the continual increase of the drugging, for as soon as the effect seems to be subsiding, more drug must be administered. It becomes a vicious circle from which there is no escape except to be sent to the ultimate end in a confused and half-deadened condition, instead of being helped to live out as many years as possible in the easiest, quietest and most gentle manner.

In his *Genius of Homœopathy*, page 79, Stuart Close gives us the following admonition :

Many substances are used medically in such form, in such doses, by such methods and upon such principles as to be distinctly depressive or destructive of normal reactivity. They are forced upon or into the suffering organism empirically without regard to nature's laws. So far as their effect upon disease is concerned they are in no wise curative, but only palliative or suppressive and the ultimate result, if it be not death, is to leave the patient in a worse state than he was before. Existing disease symptoms are transformed into the symptoms of an ·artificial drug disease. The organism is overwhelmed by a more powerful enemy which invades its territory, takes violent possession and sets up its own kingdom. Such victories over disease are a hollow mockery from the standpoint of a true therapeutics.

When we are facing these incurable conditions the administration of the similar remedy almost always ameliorates the situation, at least for three or four days, and usually for a longer period. Then we may have a return of the symptoms, when the indicated remedy will be called into use again. These conditions of impending fatality are usually accompanied by a great many symptoms, because the whole organism is involved and a gradual dissolution is taking place in every part of the economy and the vital energy is so nearly overcome as to be unable to throw off these manifestations. Sometimes one symptom or set of symptoms predominates and becomes the annoying, troublesome, disagreeable symptom-complex. In these conditions we must retake the case and re-examine the remedy that we have been using, to see if it corresponds with the disease condition. If the similarity exists in these especially troublesome manifestations, these patients can be made much more comfortable.

For instance, a recent case of incurable cancer developed involuntary urination with absolutely no control over the condition. Her remedy was one of the *Calcarea* group. For this troublesome symptom of involuntary urination the repertory gives us five remedies of equally prominent rank which we may consider : *Arsenicum, Natrum mur., Pulsatilla, Rhus tox.* and *Causticum.* With the constitutional similarity of the patient to the *Calcareas, Causticum* was the only remedy to be considered, and one dose of *Causticum* 200 restored complete control over this disagreeable symptom, and made the patient more comfortable in general.

Another class of symptoms that is very troublesome and which often falls under the use of palliatives, is composed of the patients who complain of insomnia. These patients will yield to the law of similars with pleasing results in their whole constitutional state, but not unless this symptom is considered with the concomitants that point to the remedy. Insomnia may be the outstanding irritating symptom in many varied symptom pictures. In some cases there is general coldness, and the patient will lie for hours awake unless he is covered with extra bedclothing, although he may not be aware of being uncomfortably cold. Worries of a business nature may be the cause of the accompanying symptom picture, or family disturbances may be at the bottom of the trouble. There may be pain and distress in certain parts. Any of these things attend a symptomatology of which the insomnia is but a part. Does he fall asleep if his knees are heavily covered ? Is he kept awake by a rush of ideas ? Is he lying awake because he fears that something will happen to him if he drops off to sleep ? When does he lie awake—on first going to bed or after midnight ? In other words, what are the concomitants ?

The insomnia may be treated with crude palliative measures so that the patient secures sleep, but at best this is an unnatural sleep ; while if the insomnia is considered as a part of his symptomatic picture, and given its proper place in that symptomatology and the man himself is treated —not alone one or two symptoms—he will gain his natural, refreshing sleep and he himself will be improved in general health.

Again, pain is one of the experiences from which human life has ever striven to free itself. Pain in itself is a blessing in disguise, for it brings to the patient a recognition of trouble, and to the physician the ability to recognize the location of the trouble.

The treatment of pain as a single trouble, and the fear of pain, has led to a wider use of narcotics than any other single factor. It is the cause of more drug addicts than can well be estimated. The patient is in pain, or the physician fears that the patient may be in pain, and in a sympathetic attempt to relieve the patient from a temporary discomfort many a physician has been led to prescribe drugs, the initial effect of which is to relieve the suffering of the patient, but the lasting effects of which are to produce a drug addict. Robert T. Morris, M.D., made the following statement in 1893, and it is as true to-day as it was then :

1. Opium is a drug which stupefies the physician who gives it more than it does the patient who takes it.
2. A drug which greatly relieves the distress of the physician, who, without it, would be compelled to do something rational for the relief of the patient who has put confidence in him.

Pain in itself is but a part of the symptom, however, for the physician must take into consideration the location ; the kind of pain, whether steady or intermittent, and if intermittent, whether at regular intervals or upon motion, or is it dull, cutting, blunt or sharp, pressing, pulling, darting, cramping ? Get at the type of pain as a characteristic symptom of the disordered condition ; the times and circumstances of aggravation and amelioration, the reaction to thermic conditions, and all the concomitant symptoms that can be found. When the symptom of the pain itself is complete, with the location, type, and aggravations and ameliorations, your picture is almost complete ; but if in addition you can find those concomitants (which may lie in the conditions of aggravation or amelioration but which are often from seemingly unrelated symptoms) you have a sound basis for the selection of a remedy which will relieve the pain promptly, and the patient will be much more comfortable and happy in general than with any narcotic.

One of the most difficult problems a physician has to meet, where he has need of acumen and discernment and a complete knowledge of remedy pictures, are such conditions as manifest an alternation of symptom pictures in different seasons of the year, such as summer gastric disturbances and winter rheumatic conditions, the Dr. Jekyll and Mr. Hyde of chronic manifestations. There are a number of these conditions of alternations of symptom groups, and then there are the alternation of sides. When the patient presents himself to you, you may be justified in concluding from his story that his trouble is limited to the disturbed state of which he complains at that time ; yet the remedy selected on this group of symptoms alone will often fail to bring relief, or, if the remedy does relieve the symptoms most marked at the time, the man's condition as a whole may not be improved, or indeed it may even be worse, since we have not cured but palliated a part of his symptom picture, obliterating a very valuable part of our symptomatology. If the patient is curable and we have thus obliterated a part of his symptom picture, we have blinded ourselves as to his true state; whereas a complete understanding of his condition over a period of several months would give a sound basis for a successful remedy selection. This is especially true in such conditions as gout, and we have remedies that have just this periodicity. Either for palliation of incurable diseases or for the cure of the curable diseases the symptomatology of the remedy must simulate, in so far as possible, the disease picture in order to bring relief, and where periodicity or alternation is a part of the symptomatology the remedy must have the characteristic feature if we are to expect it to be effective.

It is sometimes true, when we have a case with alternating phases or series of symptom groups and we are unable to meet the condition with a remedy that covers all the phases (either because we do not learn of the alternating phases from the patient in the first place or because we do not know of a remedy to meet the condition), that by meeting the symptom groups as they arise in the case itself as we go on, the symptomatology becomes clearer and more distinct so that we more completely meet the conditions as they arise and the patient's condition becomes better as a whole. This is meeting the case by a zigzag process, removing the most pronounced and characteristic symptoms by the remedies most similar in each state, but it takes very careful prescribing or we are apt to hopelessly mix the case. This may be done in emergencies or when we cannot find a better method. It serves better as a palliative measure in incurable states than as a curative measure in curable states, and a failure in any of one of a series of successive prescriptions may mean the difference between possibility and impossibility of eventual cure. There is far more satisfaction and the case is much more complete if we can get a picture of the whole condition and of the single remedy to meet that condition.

This may be difficult from two angles. The young physician may find it difficult to do this work carefully because he lacks the knowledge of the materia medica ; but he has at his command a wonderful source of help in his repertories, which will often serve his purpose by quick reference, filling in the knowledge that he lacks of the remedy. Another possibility is that of remedy relationships and the relationship of the various inherited dyscrasias to the case ; these are large subjects in themselves and will be discussed elsewhere. Again, it is very possible that the remedy covering the case has not been proven fully, or may not have been thought of by the students of materia medica.

Here is where the limitations of man's knowledge manifests itself. The law is correct and God-given, but no secrets of knowledge are ever given without diligent work and observation on the part of man. Much work has been done by our antecedents in developing an exceedingly valuable materia medica, and they have left a glorious record in the symptomatology of the different remedies. They have given us the weapons to meet these states ; if we fail it is not the fault of the law, nor of the weapons, but of our failure to learn the use of our equipment. Incurable cases are a source of great anxiety to every physician, but the physician who will follow the law of similars with the use of the single remedy in potentized form will give quicker relief and more sustained relief than all the massive doses of narcotics and sedatives.

In cases of mechanical injuries where there is much pain and which would be subject to narcotic or sedative treatment under ordinary medicine, the homœopathic physician has a group of vulnerary remedies that will not only allay the pain and distress incident to traumatic conditions, but will prevent congestive, suppurative or gangrenous processes and actually will hasten healing ; whereas narcotics, while deadening the pain, invite structural changes by slowing the natural recuperative powers. In this class we may mention such remedies as *Arnica, Hypericum, Ledum, Natrum sulph., Rhus tox.* and *Ruta,* each of the highest usefulness when indicated.   These remedies cannot be used successfully at random, any more than in any other condition ; but when they are similar to the condition they are of inestimable benefit.

The homœopathic physician finds another substitute for narcotics in surgical cases, either before or after operation. Here the indicated remedy does excellent service, and the patient will go through the mental and physical distress very happily.   These remedies will be indicated partly by the symptomatology of the patient and partly by the immediate cause of distress, such as lacerated wounds, strenuous vomiting, shock and incarcerated flatus.   In other words, here also the symptom must be complete.

These are the things that may be done to relieve suffering. The same law applies in curable and incurable cases, and it is very essential in curable cases that no narcotic nor hypnotic nor sedative should be used, for the reason that these cloud the whole condition ; but if the true reflection of the symptomatology be found we have a basis for help which no other means could offer.   In incurable cases, or seemingly incurable cases, we must not put a limitation on the possibilities of the similar remedy, for in many seemingly incurable conditions the *simillimum* will so completely meet the situation as to obliterate the symptomatology of disease and the pathology, and will restore the patient to health.

CHAPTER XX

TEMPERAMENTS

IN homœopathic instruction there is frequent mention of temperaments ; especially do we consider temperaments in case taking and in prescribing. Perhaps it is wise to give some consideration to a definition of temperaments, and just what weight this should have in taking the case and prescribing.

There are four classical temperaments : nervous, bilious, sanguinous, phlegmatic. There are many combinations of these types, usually with one basic type predominating. Sometimes we find people who are very difficult to classify under any type, being a combination of several basic types.

These temperaments are to a very large extent physiological, but besides the stature of the patient the matter of temperaments implies colouring, functional tendencies of circulation, elimination, respiration, and so on, and at the same time mental and emotional tendencies in reaction to environment and circumstance. The matter of temperaments is closely allied with the basic dyscrasias, which we have discussed at greater length. Our concern at this time is particularly in relation to the temperament as it has been considered an element in prescribing the homœopathic remedy.

It has been said that the temperaments are cast in the very beginning of the new individual, when the parent cells first unite, and that once cast, there is no deviation from them; and that what is physiological cannot be influenced or changed by the action of our remedies. Both these statements are to a considerable degree true, but perhaps it would be more definitely true if we said that the initial tendency cannot be changed, but that the homœopathically indicated remedy, prescribed accurately in babes and children, can so modify the physiological tendencies as to prevent their unfavourable ultimates, to a considerable degree.

The morbific influences that are attracted to temperamental tendencies are amenable to treatment and can be removed by the homœopathic remedy ; this in itself is greatly preventive of the dangers arising from temperamental weaknesses.

The homœopathic prescription is often biased by the temperament to the extent that certain temperaments bring out certain symptom pictures much more readily than do other so-called temperaments. For instance, the phlegmatic type is essentially sluggish in reaction. We expect to find venous stasis a marked tendency of this temperament, the opposite of the sanguinous. The nervous temperament, as it implies, would indicate quick action, the high strung type. In the bilious we expect to find a tendency to liver disorders. Just so far as the temperaments as classified develop symptoms in their conventional lines may we depend upon them as guides in the selection of the remedy. If we look into the case further, in the light of the hereditary dyscrasias that tend toward certain developmental changes, we will see more clearly the indications for our remedies than if we merely look at surface groupings.

We often hear patients classified on snap judgments as a *Pulsatilla* patient, a *Nux vomica* patient, or perhaps a *Phosphorus* patient, because of the general build and colouring associated with these remedies. Many mistakes have been made in prescribing on this so-called type method. Let us analyse the reasons we have for considering a phlegmatic blonde woman as a *Pulsatilla* patient. Do we mean that this colouring always indicates *Pulsatilla* ? Do we mean that a woman of this type never requires *Nux vomica* ? If we do, we have based our conclusions on a half-truth. What we really mean is that the stout young woman with blue eyes, fair hair and pale skin has developed more, and more clearly cut, symptoms under the proving than people of other colouring or stature. On the other hand, the best provers of *Nux vomica* were wiry dark men. This means that the natural physical makeup of certain people predisposing them to certain reactions under certain circumstances makes them particularly susceptible to certain disease influences, whether these disease influences are natural (created by themselves or their environment) or artificial (created by homœopathic provings). In other words, the temperament as cast in the beginning of their existence predisposes to certain morbific reactions, and, if not controlled, they will develop these reactions under certain circumstances.

On the other hand, we have not attempted the stupendous task to so classify the various elements that influence people to ascertain how people of any general type might react to any given set of circumstances that we could with assurance say that certain temperaments would develop certain symptoms. It is far simpler and easier to learn the value of the homœopathic remedy by a close study of its symptom complex, that we may recognize them in an ailing patient, and there manifest the action of the remedy as the *simillimum*.

When an individual becomes a patient, he manifests symptoms as a reaction of his inner and outer conditions and circumstances that show his susceptibility in an entirely different way than when he is in a state of equilibrium. Whereas in a state of perfect health, and therefore perfect equilibrium, he might not react at all to the introduction of a remedy, and therefore produce no symptoms, in a state of disturbed equilibrium or sickness he may develop a heightened susceptibility to the very remedy he passed by indifferently when his condition was not susceptible to its action.

Thus we may note the action of several of our frequently indicated remedies in the provings. *Belladonna* has shown marked reaction in the florid, phlegmatic temperament ; *Phosphorus* developed many symptoms in the nervous-bilious temperament ; *Baryta* reacts most effectively in the dwarfed, stunted or backward individual ; *Nux vomica* brought out the most symptoms in the nervous temperament. Certain types manifested peculiar susceptibility to certain remedies.

As the equilibrium deviates from normal it becomes more and more susceptible ; the *least possible* has an overwhelming influence in states of disturbed balance, and therefore the remedy indicated by the conditions of disturbed balance is the one that will most quickly restore the equilibrium, regardless of the temperament.

Various remedies have brought out differing provings in

different temperaments, but the recorded symptoms are useful in any temperament. Thus in the spare, narrow-chested individual the provings of *Phosphorus* produced a tubercular syndrome, while provings of the same remedy on the rotund, florid individual developed many vascular symptoms. Yet *Phosphorus* acts on all types of people, and will cure in all symptom likenesses regardless of temperamental indications. What is true of *Phosphorus* is true of every remedy in our materia medica.

It is true that the spare, narrow-chested individual that we call the *Phosphorus* type may develop *Phosphorus* symptoms more readily than a different physical stature ; but the development of symptoms according to physical makeup does not run to any proven ratio of dependability.

The indications of colouring are often considered as symptomatic. The *Pulsatilla* blonde, of whom we hear so much, is far from always requiring that remedy. The *Nux vomica* man is not always dark ; for the dark man may require *Pulsatilla* and the *Nux vomica* woman is often with us. Far more valuable than the indications of colouring or even of stature are those indications of disposition and general symptomatology, especially the modalities ; these are the true indications for our prescription. The faintness and aggravation from a close room, the amelioration from fresh open air, are far more indicative of the *Pulsatilla* patient than the blue eyes and fair skin. If we can add to these the tendency to weep and the aggravation on consolation, we may think of *Pulsatilla* with some assurance, be the patient man or woman, black or white ! As an illustration, a case of hay fever carefully repertorized left the balance divided equally between *Pulsatilla* and *Nux vomica*. The woman, red-haired, tall, vigorous, seemed to fall into neither class with any assurance on the part of the physician, so indefinite were the modalities that we expect to mark the two so clearly. Upon inquiry, however, the question of reaction to tears or anger elicited the fact that she never wept until she became thoroughly angry ; but she smouldered for some time before she got to that state. The *Nux vomica* side of the balance had the necessary additional weight, and that remedy was prescribed with remarkable success.

When a remedy is indicated, the symptomatology gives us a basis for our *simillimum* regardless of colour or type. Thus we may find a so-called woman's remedy, such as *Sepia*, distinctly indicated in a man. Some of our older teachers instructed that when a remedy was indicated out of its normal type (that is, out of the type that made the best provers of it) it was a double indication that it was needed in that particular case.

When *Pulsatilla* will develop blonde hair, or *Nux vomica* provings change the colour of the hair, the eyes, or the skin, to the true brunette type, then we may say with truth that the wiry brunette is a *Nux vomica* patient, or the blonde-haired lady is a *Pulsatilla* patient and judge them correctly at first glance.

Prescribing on types, or temperaments, is at best a slack method of using the blessings of homœopathy. It is really keynote prescribing, and then not on any morbific symptoms, but on a general stature that is present from birth. Keynotes may often give us a clue to the indicated remedy, but this clue must not be allowed to overbalance our judgment in weighing the whole symptom picture.

The only real evidence of disease conditions is the deviation from normal—the perversions of function as manifest in mind, body and spirit—the sum total of which provides us with a sound basis for prescription. The basis, then, in all of our procedure, is to find the totality of the morbific symptoms. If we find this, we can meet it through the *Law of Similars* with the single indicated potentized remedy. Then we will have cleared the patient of the morbific conditions, and will leave the personality and temperament intact and even guided into a state of healthier attractions, less liable to invasion by morbific influences.

CHAPTER XXI

LOCAL APPLICATIONS

LOCAL applications—what visions these words bring to
mind ! Mustard plasters, onion poultices, boneset and
brine—in fact, anything in common usage that could be
applied by the home nurse or procured by the most skilful
physician. From time immemorial local applications have
been the rule among the laity as domestic remedies and
among physicians from Æsculapius down to the present day.
This method of treatment was based on the teaching and
general belief that if the outward manifestations were
removed, the disease was cured ; that the outward manifestation was the disease itself, and that the individual would be
cured were the manifestations removed.

This doctrine was taught from the earliest times until
Hahnemann proclaimed to the world a new doctrine, that
the local manifestations were but an outward expression of
the inward and spiritual force, which when disturbed
expressed itself in external signs ; that if these external
manifestations were removed by local treatment, the disease
was not cured, but driven in to some more centrally
located organ, there to express itself in some graver form.

It was the custom of the older physicians to use first the
local applications ; then if the manifestation showed itself
in the internal organs, the ever-present purge was used to
drive it out. It has been said that the use of the purge was
the last remnant of pagan medicine, and was based on the
theory that all disease was caused by a very active evil spirit.

Hahnemann's teaching in regard to local applications is
very clear and distinct, and in practice has thoroughly proven
its value. *Organon*, Par. 194 :

It is neither beneficial in acute local diseases of rapid growth
nor in those of long standing, to use a remedy externally as a
local application to the diseased part, even if the medicines were

specific and curative in that form. Acute local diseases, such as inflammations of single parts, like erysipelas, for instance, which are not produced by violent external injuries, but by dynamic or internal causes, will usually yield rapidly to internal homœopathic remedies selected from our stock of well-tested medicines. . . .

In a recent homœopathic journal one of our distinguished English confréres advocated the use of the potency as a local application. This method of treatment received censorious consideration from Hahnemann, in Paragraphs 196, 197 and 198 of the *Organon*.

It may seem as if the cure of a local disease could be accelerated, not only by internal administration, but also by external application of the correct homœopathic remedy adapted to the totality of symptoms, since the effect of a medicine, applied locally to the disease itself, might possibly produce a more rapid improvement.

But this kind of treatment is entirely objectionable, not only in local affections dependent on psora, but also in local symptoms arising from syphilis and from sycosis, *because the local application of a medicine, simultaneously with its internal use, results in great disadvantages*. For in diseases characterized by a main symptom in the form of a permanent local affection, the latter is generally dispelled by topical applications more rapidly than the internal disease. This often leads to the deceptive impression that we have accomplished a perfect cure. At all events the premature disappearance of this local symptom renders it very difficult, and in some cases impossible to determine whether the total disease has also been exterminated by the internal remedy.

For the same reason, a medicine having the power of curing internally, should not be employed *exclusively as a topical application* to the local symptoms of chronic miasmatic diseases. For, if these are only topically suppressed, this partial effect will leave us in doubt regarding the action of the internal remedies, which are absolutely indispensable to the restoration of general health. . . .

What, then, should be the attitude of the Hahnemannian in regard to local applications ? Is it necessary that we leave the patient in all his discomfort in a chronic case like psoriasis and depend entirely upon the potentized remedy ? Does the intense itching necessarily prove the deciding symptom in selecting the remedy ? Just what is the meaning of local applications ? If by local applications we mean something that will thwart the expression of the disease, this certainly should not be considered beneficial according to Hahnemann's teaching ; but if we base our use of local applications upon physical principles, we may consider it. For instance, in cases of psoriasis and like diseases, the scale that is thrown off by the cuticle tears the corium. This is the cause of the intense itching and is purely a mechanical disturbance. This can be removed very easily and properly by olive oil, followed by a bathing of the part, for cleansing purposes. Such conditions as appear in erysipelas, where there is great tension and dryness, may be temporarily relieved without violating Hahnemannian principles by laying on for a few minutes a soft cloth which has been dipped in a normal salt solution. Such treatments are not local applications in the sense that Hahnemann referred to in his derogation of the practice.

There is another phase of local applications to be considered, those which have to do with the thermic reactions of the body. For instance, it would be very objectionable to put cold applications on a patient whose symptomatology calls for *Rhus tox*. It would be equally inconsistent and aggravating to put a local hot application on a *Pulsatilla* patient, and one should guard against using a hot water bottle at the feet of *Sulphur* patients. When using any adjuvants, the thermic reactions of the patient should be considered. This brings out the necessity of having a keen observation and a very thorough knowledge of the aggravations and ameliorations of our remedies, so as to avoid doing anything locally that would aggravate the general discomfort of the patient.

There is only one condition where local application of the indicated potentized remedy may be used to advantage, and that is in cases where it is impossible to administer it by mouth. This statement is based on Hahnemann's observations that mucous surfaces and denuded surfaces are receptive to the indicated remedy, but in a more limited degree than through the alimentary canal. Paragraphs 290, 291, 292 :

Besides the stomach, the tongue and mouth are the parts most susceptible of medicinal impressions ; but the lining membrane of the nose possesses this susceptibility in a high degree. Also the rectum, genitals, and all sensitive organs of our body are almost equally susceptible of medicinal effects. For this reason, parts denuded of cuticle, wounded and ulcerated surfaces, will allow the effects of medicines to penetrate quite as readily as if they had been administered by the mouth, and therefore olfaction or inhalation must be still more efficacious.

Parts of the body deprived of their natural sense, e.g. in the absence of the sense of taste or smell, the tongue, palate, and nose will impart impressions made primarily on these organs, with a considerable degree of perfection to all other organs of the body.

Also the external surface of the body, covered by the cutis and cuticle, is capable of receiving the action particularly of liquid medicines ; and the most sensitive parts of the surface are, at the same time, the most susceptible.

This is a subject which has not been made clear to many homœopathic physicians, and many well-meaning practitioners have resorted to external measures ; but there is no wavering in Hahnemann's own teaching.

There are many things in common use by physicians in general whose ultimate results need to be carefully considered by the careful physician. These methods are not confined to physicians of the regular school, but are also used by many physicians who are devoting themselves to specialties. First among these methods which are objectionable from the Hahnemannian point of view and which cause trouble for a large number of patients is the indiscriminate and persistent use of astringent sprays, which are usually permeated with medicinal ingredients. This is particularly true of nasal sprays and douches, and their action is suppressive of the natural discharges of the body whenever such treatment is used, and so clogs and shuts off the natural outlets of the sinuses in the nose and face. When the natural discharges are once suppressed and shut in, we have the ideal circumstances for abscess formation, for we have heat, moisture and bacilli. No better field can be devised, not even the incubating ovens of the laboratories.

All unnatural nose and throat discharges should be met

12

by the *simillimum* for each individual case, and it is never safe to resort to, or permit the patients to use, local means to stay the flood of discharges from the nose and throat. It is much better to let them run their course without medicine than to use the slightest means to lock the natural outlets. The satisfaction and reward that the Hahnemannian homœopath has in abiding by this rule, and staying with his patients in these aggravating conditions, and seeing them recover rapidly and painlessly in the natural order of sequence, is worth all the pains and care that are expended.

I have been in practice for nearly forty years, all of the time in New England where sinus trouble is rampant, and I have never yet had a case of sinus infection develop in my own practice. I have received many from other physicians, but have never seen one develop in a patient who has been treated with the indicated remedy.

Another field where much harm is done is in gynæcological work. Leucorrhœal discharges are exceedingly troublesome to many patients, and astringent douches are frequently ordered by specialists in this field. Lotions and astringent douches can and do suppress the quantity of these secretions, oftentimes changing their character entirely. This treatment appeals to the patient because it speedily reduces the offensiveness of the symptom. The temptation would be to do this very thing, if we did not know the fundamental law that vital energy will express itself, and in the kindliest way to the future health of the patient ; when we attempt to alter by physiological means, we are bound to disturb that vital force and cause it to express itself in some other channel than that which nature chooses.

Along this same line is the promiscuous use of local applications, deodorants to suppress or change the character of perspiration. This is exceedingly objectionable, because it leaves pent up in the system that which is poisonous and injurious to the health of the individual. This condition is not often observed by the doctor unless he by chance runs across it, or is on the alert for such suppression.

In the indiscriminate use of surgery, the habit of painting the patient with iodine is objectionable from two points— that of the absorption of the drug, and from the local irritation that this drug so frequently creates. Many patients are exceedingly susceptible to drugs in such form, and it is not uncommon for involuntary provings to be made by the local use of iodine or other applications on such a patient. One patient was particularly sensitive to zinc in any form, and felt constitutional symptoms after the use of adhesive tape or talcum powders.

I want to urge strongly the use of asepsis in our obstetrical work instead of antisepsis, because at this particular period the whole female genital tract is particularly susceptible to the use of antiseptic drugs ; whereas if asepsis is strictly carried out, the patient's recovery is uneventful.

Chapter XXII

DISEASE CLASSIFICATION

ALL scientific advancement shows epochs of great progress. In the early seventeenth century the Swedish student Linnæus studied the flora of the world, which was then largely unclassified, and through his prodigious endeavours he classified the vegetable kingdom as far as then known, and laid down a system of classification which would be applicable to further discoveries. This placed the study of botany on a scientific basis.

In 1817 and 1818 Cuvier studied the animal kingdom, the knowledge of that kingdom being at that time disjointed and unclassified. Through his stupendous labours he classified all animal life into four great kingdoms : the *Vertebrates, Mollusks, Articulates* and *Radiates.* Into these four great families all animal life can be classified.

A contemporary of Cuvier was Samuel Hahnemann. At that period, disease was known only by a few named diseases, with no relationship or method of classification. Medical practice was in an extremely chaotic condition, and was not yet free from the appellations of many years of superstition. It was still thought that diseases were the work of the evil one and no comprehensive study of disease conditions had been made. In order to establish a logical basis for the recognition of disease conditions, and their origin and relationship, it was necessary to make many close observations of the then known diseases, and then proceed to deductions and proper classifications. Hahnemann set himself to this task, bringing his logical, scientific mind to bear on the situation, and he made the first classification of diseases that had ever been attempted.

It is significant that in this endeavour he recognized the presence of bacteria and attributed to these animal forms, too minute for the eye to see, many forms of epidemic and acute illnesses ; and this deduction he announced in 1818 more than sixty years before Koch isolated the tubercle bacillus.

As Cuvier classified zoology into four great kingdoms, so Hahnemann classified disease into four great divisions. Since the principles of classification would fail unless these classifications were all-embracive, it was the work of several years to trace the course of each disease to its origin and place it in its proper classification, with due regard to its source and development.

The first of these classifications was simple, in that it embraces all diseases that might spring from mechanical and exterior sources ; this included fractures, strains, indiscretions of diet, external poisons such as fumes or noxious plants, extremes of thermic conditions such as frostbite or sunstroke, and all trade diseases. This class embraced conditions which are largely self-curative in that they may be rectified by regulating environment and habits.

While these conditions may be self-curative if the conditions are regulated, medicine may assist and hasten the recovery. Any of the conditions in this classification may be more or less mixed with more deep-seated conditions from another and deeper origin, and this may so complicate the matter that medicine will be required to alleviate the resultant distress.

Repeated claims have been made that the followers of Hahnemann treat diseases by the symptoms only, applying remedies according to the symptomatology and paying attention only to the symptomatic applicability of remedies ; but it cannot be emphasized too strongly that Hahnemann made one classification of disease conditions that were dependent entirely on external causes, such as the mechanical conditions. It was Hahnemann's teaching that the removal of the cause was the first step in the proper method of cure. This may occasion at times surgical procedure ; rectification of diet ; the removal of irritating substances ; change of environment ; anything and everything that may place the patient in the best possible relation for complete cure, which will take place of itself when the cause is removed.

Hahnemann taught by precept and example the value of thinking through to the beginning, the first cause, of disease conditions, and treating them accordingly.

In his observation of cases, and in the further study of the progress of diseased conditions under the homœopathic method of treatment, Hahnemann was especially struck with the course of non-venereal diseases. Hahnemann found himself treating seemingly acute conditions with apparent success, but, to his surprise, these cases would return with a recurrence of symptoms at intervals ; sometimes these symptoms were very similar to those they had had before, while at other times there would be an aggravation of the previous condition, or other variations. Considerable study of these cases convinced Hahnemann that there was some underlying condition which was the mainspring of these recurrent manifestations and which was causing more or less gradually a retrograde condition, although the acute manifestations were apparently met and conquered by the homœopathic remedy. It occurred to him that he was treating in these acute conditions only a part of the real disease ; otherwise the disease would have become completely and permanently cured by the administration of the *simillimum.*

If these exacerbated symptoms were but a fragment of the disease, then there must be a much deeper, primitive force underlying these sporadic manifestations, which could be judged only by the force and frequency of the reappearance. It became Hahnemann's study to take into consideration these deeper conditions from which sprang the acute diseases, as a part of the prescription necessary to cure. It was his aim to find a remedy which would meet the acute condition and the presumably hidden condition at the same time. In order to undertake this stupendous task it was necessary to study a vast number of cases and to consider and develop a number of remedies to meet his requirements, and find a remedy which was to cure both the acute symptoms and the underlying chronic sickness; to conquer the hidden primitive malady.

This involved two lines of investigation, one in natural chronic disease conditions and one in artificially produced

disease conditions which should be similar in symptomatology
and depth of action to the natural disease.

In his study of disease, he separated all disease conditions
into the four great groups before mentioned. The
mechanical conditions were easily detected and classified.
To the three remaining groups Hahnemann gave the term
miasms.

The manifestations of chronic disease conditions which
Hahnemann called *miasms* were so designated by him for
want of a better term ; in fact, in the German language and
in Hahnemann's day the word *miasm* properly defined the
idea Hahnemann had in mind. In the development of
modern diagnostic terms, and in the English language of
to-day, this designation seems to be out of place and a
word of explanation is needed.

According to the common definition, a miasm is defined
as *polluting exhalations or malarial poisons*. It is obvious
that the word in English does not interpret intelligently
Hahnemann's meaning. Therefore, the residual poisons of
syphilis and gonorrhœa that have become, according to
Hahnemann's classification, the *miasms of syphilis and
sycosis*, might better be termed the *stigmata of syphilis and
gonorrhœa*. The effect of either virus affecting the primordial
cell casts a stigma or blight upon the developing cell that is
nearly ineffaceable. The same stigma may be laid upon the
constitution of an individual by acquiring the disease, if the
virus is not thoroughly eradicated from the system.

The word *sycosis*, coming from the Greek word meaning
fig, has found a place in the modern medical dictionary with
several definitions, one of which is as follows : *Hahnemann's
term for the constitutional effects of the gonorrhœal virus*. Thus
we see that one of the accepted definitions of the word
sycosis is that which Hahnemann had in mind, and which he
called alternatively the *fig wart disease*.

In many instances it was very easy for him to trace the
venereal relationship of disease conditions, and he soon found
it easy to recognize the branding of this group. At first he
classed these under one head, but later divided the venereal
miasms into two classifications, *syphilis* and *sycosis*, or
gonorrhœa.

PSORA

However, the great majority of disease conditions remained unclassified. For ten years cases were studied, patients were closely questioned, and even history was called upon to divulge the course of diseases through the centuries. Through endless difficulties Hahnemann traced these hitherto unclassified diseases, and gave to them the name of *psora*. This word *psora*, which Hahnemann used to denote the third great miasm, is defined by the modern medical dictionary as follows :

1. *Scabies.* 2. *Psoriasis.* 3. *Hahnemann's term for the " itch dyscrasia ", defined as the parent of all chronic diseases—skin diseases, neoplasms, insanity, etc.; it was similar to, though of more extended application than, the " herpeti diathesis " of French writers.* And the definition adds : *p. leprosa, psoriasis.*

Funk & Wagnall's *Dictionary* gives : *Psora.* 1. *Pathol. The itch, or some such similar skin disease.* 2. *The itch mite.* The derivation is Latin and Greek, but it is rather Hebraic in origin, coming through the Greek and Latin, the original word being *tsorat*.

Interpretation of this Hebrew word *tsorat* conveys clearly the thought Hahnemann had in mind. *Tsorat : A groove, a fault ; a pollution ; a stigma ; often applied to leprous manifestations and to the great plagues.* It is the meaning of the original Hebrew word that we must regard as the basis for the term covering this constitutional defect.

In the light of modern comprehension of these conditions, classified by Hahnemann as psora, we may not doubt but that the original meaning of the Hebrew word had greater significance than we have understood. *A groove, a fault.* . . . With our growing knowledge of the so-called deficiency diseases we are coming to realize that the lack of certain elements in the system, or the inability to assimilate them from foods, is the great common denominator of almost all the so-called psoric conditions, plus a lack of balance in the equilibrium of health that manifests through a hypersensitivity of impressions—functional disturbances and the patient's recognizance of disturbance that varies from consciousness to neuroses.

The vast majority of the diseases of the earth came under this great classification, which has been called the mother of all diseases; and Hahnemann found that there was a traceable relationship between these chronic manifestations and the many various plagues which had troubled the peoples of the earth since the most ancient times, manifesting themselves in various ways, such as the ancient plagues of Egypt, leprosy (at one time France alone had over two thousand homes for lepers), and the itch poison which swept Europe at a later date. In many instances Hahnemann found there was a close connection between such grave infectious diseases and the patients with stubborn recurring symptoms.

Hahnemann became convinced that these recurring symptoms owed their existence to this chronic miasm which he called psora, and that of itself this condition could never be cured. While the acute manifestations may subside and be quiescent for a considerable period, the chronic state that causes the acute eruption of symptoms never dies until it is met with the similar remedy.

Hahnemann found that this form of disease was first made manifest on the skin, as a skin infection or eruption; this was its natural place, but here the natural manifestation is susceptible of suppression by many forms of treatment, such as lotions, ointments, mineral baths, surgical operations with the removal of organs, and anything that tends to obliterate the manifestation on the surface by seemingly curing the external symptoms. It is on the surface that it naturally thrives and here it will do the least harm. By suppression this constitutional state becomes more manifest in a train of distressing symptoms, so long as the skin manifestation is quiescent, and may affect any part of the body.

Hahnemann found, too, that many chronic ailments which are enumerated in pathological works under distinct names, originate, with few exceptions, in this widely ramified psora. All skin manifestations and conditions; almost all adventitious formations such as swelling of the glands, sarcomatous and carcinomatous tumours; deformed bony structures; hæmorrhagic tendencies; all suppurations;

functional disturbances; nutritional disturbances; all of the acute disease manifestations; all these conditions Hahnemann traced to this source and classified under the head of psora.

It is characteristic of the skin in these conditions that there is considerable itching, for psoric conditions always itch. In fact, not only was psora considered the mother of all diseases, but it might well have been considered as the source of almost all subjective symptoms, especially those described by the patient " sensation as if ". In classifying those constitutional diseases which have not run a course through so many centuries, that is, the venereal classifications, it has been noted that their action has been swifter, and while at times more destructive, the subjective symptoms have been present *in the degree in which psora has been present in the system.*

Although fundamental miasms have their period of remission, latent states lasting perhaps for years without showing any manifestations, some sudden crisis in the history of the individual may rouse them to sudden eruption and the patient will become severely disturbed in health. These crises may be in the form of accidents, exposure, some slight infection, indiscretions of diet or hygiene, some apparently simple thing out of all proportion to the serious consequences. In this class come the pneumonias following accidents and exposures; infections from slight wounds; almost all of those grave states roused by a seemingly slight cause.

Here the homœopathic physician, by taking into consideration the psoric background, will bring into play the remedies that are related in their symptomatology to these psoric states, and he will be able to do most effective work.

The development of the similar remedy to meet these conditions led Hahnemann to understand the real nature of disease. He realized that it was the dynamic force of the remedy that met the dynamic force of disease, and that the remedy must meet the disease on the dynamic plane, but that the drug dynamis must be more potent than the disease dynamis if the disease were to be eradicated.

The action of the stigma is to debilitate the life force, to deform the body, to dull the intellect and to upset reason.

The miasms are destructive in every way, of both the mind and the body, and they tear at the very spirit of man. It is disorganizing disease that fills the state institutions of every description, and we cannot meet these conditions intelligently until we recognize the ancient origin of disease and undertake its extermination on the basis of the miasms.

To classify disease conditions as circumstantial or environmental is to view them in a limited way, and we must recognize the background and meet them on that ground if we are to cure. For this reason it is essential to find the *simillimum*, and to find the remedy for these conditions we must seek a deep-acting remedy—call it an antipsoric if you will—to eradicate the evil. It is only by using the dynamic form of the *simillimum* that we can hope to eradicate the evil.

In fact, only the dynamic form of the similar remedy can possibly be the *simillimum* for these cases, since these chronic conditions are so closely knit with every fibre of the patient's being that they have influenced his innermost dynamis. So no matter how like the symptomatology of the remedy to that of the patient, unless the remedy is in a dynamic form it cannot reach the basic stigma.

Chapter XXIII

DISEASE CLASSIFICATION : PSORA, continued

Psora has numerous sensations of vertigo. These are of many kinds and accompany all kinds of motion, and are often induced or aggravated by emotional disturbances. Hahnemann speaks of the vertigos of psora as being many and peculiar, brought on by walking, motion, looking up quickly, rising from sitting or lying ; bilious vertigo, floating, from digestive disturbances, with specks before the eyes ; desire to keep quiet by lying down, which > . In this desire to lie down and > by lying down we have the outstanding characteristic of the whole underlying condition.

There are sharp, severe, paroxysmal headaches which come on in the morning, increase as the sun rises and > when the sun goes down. These are usually frontal, temporal or parietal. The headaches with red face, throbbing, > • by rest, quiet and sleep and > by hot applications are psoric.

The bilious nausea and vomiting, coming on at regular intervals, > from rest, quiet and sleep, are psoric.

The characteristic desire to lie down and be quiet is manifest in feverish children, who desire only to be let alone.

Psoric manifestations may be a link in almost all disease conditions, and they are always > by heat.

Psora alone never causes structural changes, and the psoric head is normal in size and contour. The hair and scalp are dry, rarely perspiring ; the hair is lustreless and so dry that it cannot be combed without wetting the comb. The hair falls out after an illness. It becomes grey too early, or white in spots ; it breaks and the ends split. The skin and scalp appear unclean, and there is much itching dandruff and dry eruptions on the scalp, either papular or eczematous, which itch. These eruptions are < in the open air, < evenings ; > by scratching, but burning and smarting follow the scratching. These eruptions do not suppurate but dry down and become dead scales.

There are many eye symptoms, but since there are no structural changes under this uncomplicated stigma, we find no pathological changes. The symptoms all have to do with the functional relationships and are closely related to emotional disturbances. The psoric eye is intolerant of daylight or sunlight, and the symptoms are < in the morning, from the rising of the sun to the zenith, and > by heat. There are spots before the eyes ; this is a characteristic manifestation of this miasm, or stigma.

Ptosis of the lids is never psoric, but syphilitic. Red lids are a combination of the psoric and syphilitic in the tubercular diathesis.

The ear troubles, like the eye troubles, are functional or nervous. The appearance of the ear is normal ; the ear is small or medium in size, and never transparent in appearance. There is no moisture in or about the ear, as with the other miasms. The auditory canal is dry and scaly. We rarely find an abscessed condition in the psoric ear. Since this stigma has such marked nervous reflexes, we expect to find the characteristic oversensitiveness to sounds.

The shape of the psoric face is that of an inverted pyramid, but the face and head do not perspire as does the syphilitic condition. Perspiration is characteristic also of the tubercular diathesis, but this is because of the syphilitic admixture with the psoric. The lips are red, often red to bluish, parched and dry. The usual feverish face in the psoric patient is red and hot and shining. There are the characteristic dry itching pimples and simple acne. The skin is naturally dry, with an unwashed appearance. Rushes of blood to the face or burning of hands or feet are psoric, as are hot flushes at the climacteric.

In the nose also we find the oversensitiveness to odours ; unusual odours awaken him from sleep ; he cannot sleep where there are strong odours ; perfumes make him feel ill and faint. There are painful boils or pimples on the septum, but no malignant manifestations.

Lupus of the nose is a manifestation of the combined stigmata, and closely allied to tuberculosis.

Sordes about the mouth are psoric manifestations. There is swelling and burning about the lips rather than fissures. There is thrush and stomatitis in the mouth. The psoric patient has many taste perversions ; there is a bad taste in the mouth ; or it may be sweet, bitter or sour ; there is a regurgitation of the taste of foods ; these patients are very sensitive to taste. While all the miasms, or stigmata, have many perversions of taste, psora is the only one which manifests the symptom of burnt taste.

Psora is always hungry ; this miasm has desires and longings for many and various things. They are hungry even with the stomach full ; they are never satisfied even while eating. They crave sweets, acids, sour things ; in fevers they crave indigestible things. They long for travel, yet they are weak and debilitated ; they long for things the system is wanting ; they long for certain things, but when the want is gratified they do not want them. During pregnancy they long for peculiar things ; yet after gestation they loath the things they have craved. Before bilious attacks they crave sweets, but the attack is not caused by the sweets they consume ; rather the craving is a forerunner of the attack, a prodromal symptom.

There is a weak, gone feeling in the stomach in the middle of the forenoon ; hunger at night also is a prominent symptom. These patients lack the power of assimilation, which is undoubtedly the cause of the continual craving, and is closely related to the characteristic gnawing in the stomach with sensations of heat and cold. There is a repugnance to boiled foods ; they crave fried and highly seasoned foods, meats and greasy foods, but these do not suit. Meats stimulate the psoric patient and arouse the underlying condition to activity. In fevers they have an aversion to sweets and crave acids. The sense of fullness, gas, bloating, etc., are markedly psoric traits, and they are accompanied by heartburn and waterbrash. Most of the aggravations of psora occur after eating.

The cravings and longings are basic phenomena of great therapeutic value. A comparison of the desires of the stigmatic influences is of much help in selecting the remedy : psora desires hot foods ; syphilis prefers cold food ; sycosis wants the food either hot or cold. Psora desires meats, but the combination of psora and syphilis, in the tubercular diathesis, has an aversion to meats.

With the bloating of the psoric patient, he cannot endure the slightest touch on the abdomen ; he fears even the slightest contact.

While pure psora does not produce any structural changes, psora does produce functional changes ; these are manifest in the chest condition by the anæmic manifestations that have their effect on the duty of furnishing oxygen for the red blood cells. The emotional reaction of psora hampers the natural functions to such an extent that the functions are disturbed and the oxygen circulation feels the lack of the vitalizing influence.

The coughs of psora are dry, teasing, spasmodic and annoying. The expectoration is usually mucous, scanty, tasteless. The salty and sweetish taste of the expectoration are dependable indications of the combined psoric and syphilitic taints.

In the heart there are functional disturbances with violent rushes of blood to the chest, and a sensation of weakness, goneness or fullness about the heart. The sensation as of a band is psoric. This miasm, or stigma, manifests its reflex relationship of gastric or uterine irritations by marked palpitations or sensations as of hammering about the heart. With the heart symptoms there is always anxiety and fear on the part of the patient. The psoric patient always fears that he will die from heart trouble ; but the psoric patient is the chronic who lives long and produces income for the physician, for he is the victim of so many unpleasant sensations that he requires much attention, and his habit of fixing his attention upon one or more organs as being the cause of his discomfort demands constant attendance from the physician. He does have many uncomfortable sensations, such as sharp cutting neuralgic pains about the heart. These patients think they are about to die and want to lie down and keep quiet, but there is no danger ; it is the sycotic and syphilitic heart patients who die, and then suddenly and without warning. The psoric heart conditions are very much influenced by strong emotions, joy, grief, fear, and so on. These conditions are < eating and drinking ; there are palpitations and eructations of large amounts of gas ; sometimes the pulsations of the heart will shake the whole body. The psoric patient is always conscious of his heart condition, and it is he who is constantly taking his own pulse.

Psora alone produces more marked anasarca and dropsical conditions than sycosis. The sycotic patient succumbs before the dropsical condition becomes marked ; but the union of these two stigmata produces these conditions in a marked degree.

The abdomen feels full after eating ; there is much distension, < in the morning. The muscles are flabby, and all abdominal pains are > by heat.

The diarrhœas of psora are often induced by overeating. The patient is always hungry and eats beyond his capacity and upsets his digestive powers. This overeating often produces a colic and watery diarrhœa, usually in the morning. These diarrhœas fit the symptomatology of such remedies as *Aloe*, *Podophyllum*, and *Sulphur*, among others.

In the tubercular diathesis there is also the morning < of the diarrhœa, and the tubercular condition shows its psoric parentage by the < from cold.

Psora has a spasmodic offensive and painless diarrhœa which usually > the suffering, but it is not a persistent diarrhœa ; it comes on from emissions or from preparations for an unusual event ; after taking cold ; < by cold ; > hot drinks or heat in general.

There is a stubborn, marked, persistent constipation, with small, hard, difficult stools and no desire for stool ; or there may be alternation of the constipation and diarrhœa. With the constipation there are frequently accompanying troubles in other parts of the organism, or seemingly unrelated symptoms which are actually concomitants.

Psora is not only the mother of all diseases, but it is the psoric element which gives the valuable concomitant symptoms and furnishes the modalities and sensations which are a true expression of their sufferings. The psoric patients suffer considerably, probably much more than in the other stigmata, and with less apparent cause.

In children afflicted with this underlying condition we find retention of the urine whenever the body gets chilled, and this condition arises in old people also. An opposite indication of the psoric stigma is the involuntary urination when sneezing, coughing or laughing. There is smarting and burning on urination, but not from pathological causes. Many symptoms of this stigma are reflected in the sexual sphere, especially in women. In other words, these are functional disturbances closely related to the emotions, and dysmenorrhœa, amenorrhœa, and many other conditions result. Hahnemann tells us that grief or sorrow, such as that caused by an unhappy marriage, will produce more serious and distressing symptoms in the psoric patient than the most unfavourable surroundings or real hardships. It can be seen that there would be a marked reaction on the functions which are so closely related to the nervous system. The psoric skin is dry, rough, dirty or unhealthy appearing. In fact, the classic psoric remedy is *Sulphur*, although it is not to be thought that *Sulphur* will cure all cases nor is it limited in its range of applicability to psoric conditions ; but if there is any one remedy which we may limit by saying that it is the picture of a stigma, we may truly say that psora and *Sulphur* are so like each other, in many instances, that each typifies the other. In appearance, the psoric patients are the " great unwashed " ; bathing is unwelcome and < the roughness of the skin and the irritability.

In all psoric conditions, itching is a persistent symptom. There is very little suppuration ; there may be a few vesicles or a papular manifestation. Psoric eruptions are not noticeable by their colour, but by the roughness of the skin. Unless there is marked inflammation they are the same colour as the skin. With the dry skin, there is a decided tendency for fine, thin scales ; the eruptions dry down and scale off.

Erysipelatous manifestations are a combination of psora and sycosis.

If there is any syphilitic taint in combination with the psoric base, the patients are very apt to be susceptible to impetigo, for this is the soil in which impetigo flourishes ; without these united taints a patient will not become infected with impetigo.

13

F - 13A

The psoric patient has the symptom of coldness associated with even slight ailments ; with headaches there is a deadly coldness that is almost worse than the headache itself, and this is much < by continued effort and > by lying down where it is warm and quiet.

Modern medicine tells us that migraine has as its underlying cause emotional disturbances. In other words, this is a verification of Hahnemann's teaching on the disturbances roused in the psoric patient by grief, sorrow or other harrowing emotions.

It kills the psoric patient to stand still ; he must walk instead of standing, even if he is on his feet but a brief time. He may stand if he can lean against anything sufficiently to take the weight off his feet. This is not because of structural changes ; it is because of his natural desire to rest, with his characteristic restlessness. Weakness of the ankle joints is a sure indication of the presence of a syphilitic taint in combination with the psoric stigma.

CHAPTER XXIV

PSORA OR DEFICIENCY ?

CRITICISM of Hahnemann's psora theory has raged for a century. It is not feasible to follow minutely Hahnemann's line of reasoning that led to his declaration of the psora theory, but we have his own statement that it took years to classify what he came to term the psoric miasm. Enough has been written to show that his reasoning in this respect was sound, and as far as it went, clear. It is not strange that in the light of modern knowledge new arguments have arisen to assail this theory. Let us examine it in the light of present-day knowledge.

We have considered the general symptomatology forming the psoric group. Now let us turn to Bœnninghausen's list of antipsoric remedies, and try to prove our problem along the same lines we should employ were we to prove a problem in arithmetic. This list, comprising fifty remedies, was published in Hahnemann's time, and has been used with remarkable success in the so-called psoric conditions from that time forward :

Agaricus	*Causticum*	*Magnesium mur.*
Alumina	*Clematis*	*Manganum*
Ammonium carb	*Colocynth*	*Mezereum*
Ammonium mur.	*Conium*	*Muriatic acid*
Anacardium	*Digitalis*	*Natrum carb.*
Arsenicum alb.	*Dulcamara*	*Natrum mur.*
Aurum	*Euphorbium*	*Kali nit.*
Baryta carb.	*Graphites*	*Nitric acid*
Belladonna	*Guaicum*	*Petroleum*
Bor. ac.	*Hepar sulph.*	*Phosphorus*
Bovista	*Iodine*	*Phosporic acid*
Calcarea carb	*Kali carb.*	*Platinum*
Carbo animalis	*Lycopodium*	*Rhododendron*
Carbo veg.	*Magnesium carb.*	*Sarsaparilla*

Senega	*Stannum*	*Sulphuric acid*
Sepia	*Strontium*	*Zincum*
Silica	*Sulphur*	

Sixteen of the remedies listed belong definitely to the vegetable group, one definitely to the animal group ; of the remaining thirty-three remedies, comprising the chemical elements or inorganic substances, or combined from these elements or substances (or reduced to almost elemental consideration, as the *Carbo's*) we find only three (*Baryta, Platinum* and *Aurum*) *that appear in the range of chemical elements higher by atomic weight than those essential to the construction of the human body.* The three remedies having their source in the higher-than-body construction elements may be considered as falling into the antisyphilitic class, and we may reasonably question their adaptability to the antipsoric condition when unmixed with a venereal taint.

Let us set aside for the time these three which seem to us questionably allocated to this group, and proceed with our hypothesis.

Some thirty elements, more or less, have been ascertained by different investigators as appearing in the human body. It has been definitely established that many of these are absolutely essential to physical construction. Iodine, number 53 of the elements, is regarded as the highest in atomic weight ; and as we have pointed out, only the three that we have questioned appear in the antipsoric list beyond iodine.

The following list of elements appearing in the human body has been compiled from several sources. It is notable that not all these elements have been assigned constructive roles, in the eyes of investigators ; or rather, their presence in the body structure has not been determined. Nevertheless, all these come within the first fifty-three elements, as determined by atomic weight.

1. Hydrogen.	11. Sodium.	17. Chlorine.
3. Lithium.	12. Magnesium.	19. Potassium.
6. Carbon.	13. Aluminium.	20. Calcium.
7. Nitrogen.	14. Silicon.	22. Titanium.
8. Oxygen.	15. Phosphorus.	25. Manganese.
9. Fluorine.	16. Sulphur.	26. Iron.

27. Cobalt.   30. Zinc.   35. Bromine.
28. Nickel.   32. Germanium.   50. Tin.
29. Copper.   33. Arsenic.   53. Iodine.

Morse tells us (*Applied Biochemistry*) :

It is seen that no inert element, like argon,* occurs in the body ; that radioactive elements and those that are undergoing decomposition are lacking ; and that with regard to atomic weight, iodine is the farthest up the scale. Heavy elements, such as lead, and the noble metals, are not found. Two explanations may be offered :

(1) The distribution of the elements in the human organism is an historical matter, representing the period in evolution when only those elements that are of lighter weight than iodine were evolved. This is not probable.

(2) The lighter kinds occurring in living things because these elements were relegated to the surface of the earth and were available for the use of the organism as it has undergone evolution. The geologist believes that the heavier elements lie toward the centre of the earth, since the total weight of the earth demands heavier substances near the centre of the mass.

So in reality we might add to our list argon (18) and nitrogen (7) as appearing with some regularity in the body. With our knowledge of the power of the infinitesimals beyond the range of laboratory analysis we dare not say that any element, however small its portion or vague its relationship, " plays no part ".

Again, with our knowledge of the disturbing powers of the radio-active elements, we can see definitely why they were not included in construction, for they are essentially destructive. These correspond to the action of the syphilitic taint, and should be classed as anti-syphilitic in action.

However, we are discussing primarily those elements which, in simple form or combined, are essentially constructive, to demonstrate the significance of our hypothesis that *Psora*, and *Deficiency in properly balanced essentials, are one and the same* ; or if they are not identical problems, we must admit that here lies a significant key to the problem of psora, and one worthy of deeper study.

* Argon accompanies air into the lungs as nitrogen does, but in both cases they play no part in the economy of the body.

Without question there is some essential failure of the system to assimilate the necessary constructive materials that provides the background of the so-called psoric taint ; yet we find that emotional or other stress develops the psoric symptomatology even in constitutions that have been sound and healthy. Here we find that our theory of psora as a deficiency of the proper elements is verified. For instance, those chest conditions with many functional symptoms : we are often able to trace these to improper breathing habits, and this again to emotional strain that has broken the habit of rhythm ; or perhaps the breathing habit has been normal until the necessity of remaining long hours in close, unaired rooms has forced the system to unnatural and insufficient intake of oxygen.

The greatest asset of the body is that of adaptability, but this in itself, under unnatural or forced conditions, while permitting life to continue under emergent or hampered conditions, breeds a train of symptoms that Hahnemann described as psoric.

The body elements best known to the student of bio-chemistry are : Hydrogen, Oxygen, Carbon, Nitrogen, Fluorine, Sodium, Magnesium, Silicon, Phosphorus, Sulphur, Chlorine, Potassium, Calcium, Manganese, Iron, Copper, Zinc, Arsenic and Iodine. Chemists have been able to estimate the percentage of these elements present in the organism, even such small amounts as those of arsenic, with its sixth-decimal proportions in thyroid and brain, and 0·000,001,9 per cent. in the liver. It is comparatively easy to define the constructive purposes of many of these elements, such as calcium ; yet there is some purpose aside from that of mere bricks-and-mortar for even the most obvious. Magnesium is found throughout the body, in the lungs, glands, brain, muscles and muscular organs such as the heart. This has been determined with a fair amount of measurable accuracy ; yet how do we account for the fact that a magnesium-free diet sends animals into convulsions ? Or that tin, found in traces in the tongue and brain, is related definitely to the sense of taste ? When cobalt and nickel, discovered in the pancreas, are lacking, just what influence does this have in the development of diabetes ?

Manganese is an accompaniment of iron in practically all human tissue. Scientists have discovered that manganese starvation in animals will produce sterility in the male and loss of mother-love in the female ; this loss of maternal instinct incites them to refuse attention to their young, who die in a few hours. McCollum tells us : " When to the carefully prepared manganese-free diet is added as little as five-thousandths of 1 per cent. of manganese, all the abnormalities described are corrected." Yet Reiman and Minot tell us : " Prolonged feeding of moderate amounts of its ores to dogs failed to produce significant changes in the manganese content of the blood and tissues or to cause any pathological symptoms."

It is comparatively easy to determine the broader outlines of the constructive duties of these elements and inorganic substances, but it is the subtle and potential influences (as illustrated by the observations on manganese) that are most pertinent to our thesis. In other words, it is not the over-feeding or gross starvation of any element that provides us with the so-called psoric problem, but the subtle functional disturbance with many sensations. It is in this subtler sphere that we find the connection between the constructive essentials and the so-called antipsoric remedies. Since the so-called psoric conditions are largely functional and react pre-eminently upon the nervous and emotional plane, may we not regard these conditions as a lack of balance in the ability to assimilate, as well as a possible starvation of essentials ?

In a comparison of the constructive role of these substances (as determined by laboratory technique) with their more subtle manifestations (demonstrated through provings of the homœopathic potentiations), let us look again at manganese :

Reiman and Minot (*J. Biological Chemistry*) " found it to be present in practically all human tissue, the liver carrying more than any other " ; J. H. Clarke (*Dictionary of the Materia Medica*) cites its ability to produce inflammation and fatty degeneration of the liver. We have seen its association with iron in the blood. and homœopathically, it has its place in anæmic conditions when indicated. We have noted the laboratory observation of the loss of maternal instinct.

Clarke gives as the first mental symptom : Peevishness and taciturnity, with concentration in self." Sterility has not been a proven symptom, yet Clarke gives : " Sensation of weakness in (male) genital organs."

Speaking of the necessity for carbohydrates in the diet, McCollum (*Food, Nutrition and Health*) says :

During digestion and absorption through the intestinal walls all of these (forms of carbohydrates) are converted into glucose. Glucose is the one sugar which always occurs in the blood. Although it is present in blood only to the extent of one part per thousand of blood, this sugar is the principal fuel which is burned by the muscles for providing energy for keeping the body warm and for muscular work.

Carbohydrates are the usual form in which carbon, the element, is found in the system and in which it is ingested. This is the physiological sphere ; now let us turn to the role the carbons occupy in the list of antipsoric remedies. In Bœnninghausen's list we find *Ammonium carb.*, *Baryta carb.*, *Calcarea carb.*, *Carbo animalis*, *Carbo veg.*, *Graphites*, *Kali carb.*, *Magnesium carb.*, *Natrum carb.*, *Sepia* ; all these have the characteristic carbon influence, even though associated with another element. It may seem strange to the casual student of materia medica to include *Sepia* in this list, but to the homœopathician *Sepia* is the animal carbon.

In spite of our belief that *Barium* belongs pre-eminently to the antisyphilitic group, *Baryta carb.* bears the family relationship of the carbons, which admits it to the antipsoric, or deficiency, group as well. *Carbo an.* and *Carbo veg.* manifest most markedly the characteristic homœopathic indications for their use : *burned out* defines the condition in one word. This burned out energy and its end-results of lack of body heat and muscular strength extends even into the mental sphere ; and whether it comes from excesses, loss of animal fluids, from emotional, mental or physical stress, it is the red thread that runs all through the proven symptoms of the carbon combinations. This symptomatic thread runs all through the various spheres of action of each individual remedy of the carbon family, mental, moral, and all the varying physical fields in which it is applicable—and inasmuch as it is found in its physiological form throughout the system, so we find its symptomatology running through every part.

Calcium is an essential of bony structure and is a necessary, small but constant, essential of the blood. The homœopathic materia medica indicates the *Calcarea* group in " scrofulous " conditions ; rickety children ; large heads with open fontanelles ; and a host of symptoms we have already described in those conditions traceable to psora. McCollum tells us that calcium in the food is not enough : " Human infants often develop rickets when receiving a sufficiency of calcium and phosphorus provided they are deprived of sunlight and vitamin D."

This last comment, *provided they are deprived of sunlight* . . . leads us to meditate upon that comment of Hahnemann in relation to psora, to the effect that unnatural or unhappy surroundings are extremely dangerous to the vital energy.

It is not necessary to compare the symptomatology of many of our remedies with the body elements to bear out our contention that the problems of psora and deficiency are closely related. Any thoughtful student may verify further comparisons in the homœopathic materia medica.

In these days one rarely has the opportunity to see a patient released from emotional and economic stress into simple and natural surroundings, with much outdoor life and a simple, natural food supply free from adulterations and replete with the stored elements direct from Nature's lavish supply. However, if such a case is observed, one learns many things about the resilience of the human economy under the proper conditions. It leads one to a different outlook upon psora and its relation to the undue stress of modern life and economic conditions. We have stated repeatedly that emotional strain was an important factor in developing psoric conditions : the inability to relax for the natural and important functions demanded by Nature. Hustle and bustle take away our rhythmic, full, deep breathing ; the hurry for trains and timeclocks interferes too often with the excretory functions ; the demands of society lead us to suppress natural perspiration ; anxiety over almost every item of our lives gets in its dangerous work and often deprives us of necessary rest—certainly of chance moments of relaxation.

All these circumstances pressing upon a delicate adjustment of spirit, mind and body (especially if this be predisposed by inheritance to maladjustment) cannot but make confusion worse confounded. And at this point, if we pass on to our unborn children our inhibitions and suppressions of the spirit, mind and flesh, what can we expect but to build for them a future lacking the ability to receive from natural sources those elements—not always measurable nor as yet defined—that are essential to health ? And when we ponder that wrong living conditions, appalling plagues and seasons of famine have been cyclic since History began, we cannot wonder at an inherited tendency to disease that Hahnemann called psoric.

Whether this tendency to the psoric manifestations develops because of inability to assimilate or inability to relax to the point of assimilation, the end-results are the same, and will continue to be until corrected through more healthy and natural ways of living plus the power of the potentized remedy to release suppressions and tune the maladjustments to order.

Chapter XXV

SOME MANIFESTATIONS OF LATENT PSORA

In the last chapter you learned something of the acute manifestations of the psoric stigma. Besides the manifestations of the acute diseases, which are all directly traceable to the eruptions of psora, the vital energy often places the psoric poison in a latent state, where it may lie for a long period, sometimes for years, without manifesting much disturbance, except that the observant physician may read its peculiar characteristics, even in that latent state, and even though the patient is not disturbed to any degree.

During this latent state it requires only a slight shock to the vital energy to bring this miasm, or stigma, to the fore and make its presence actively manifest in an acute disturbance. This acute manifestation may be due to any one of many different causes ; it may be due to an accident, to an exposure, or to any other seemingly slight cause ; but whatever the direct cause of the acute manifestation, it will show the poisonous effects of the stigma, and it is well for the physician to be conversant with the characteristics of the latent state so that he may cure the underlying dyscrasia in the latent condition and thus head off the acute manifestations, thus protecting the resistant power of the vital energy against the sudden strain and helping to eradicate the psoric poison.

One of the strongest characteristics of psora in its latent state is the mental condition. Psoric patients are mentally alert ; they are quick and active in their motions. This activity is very pronounced, and especially pronounced is the keenness and activity of the mind. They will work like Trojans for a short time, but they are easily fatigued, both mentally and physically, and a profound prostration follows. This prostration has such a profound effect upon them that they soon come to the pass where they dread to undertake any exertion, mental or physical, because of the fatigue which they know will follow. The fatigue is accompanied by the desire to lie down, and this desire is quite characteristic of this type of patient.

A peculiar characteristic of the mental irritation is that it produces a sense of bodily heat, and these patients will have flushes of heat while they are working. The heat of the room oppresses them.

Another peculiarity of the mental state is anxiety. This symptom is written all over them ; they are anxious to the point of worry and fear : fear that they will be unable to accomplish what they attempt ; that they will not be able to carry through their plans ; fear that their health will fail in doing what they set out to do. If they get sick they fear death, or that they will be incurable, and they become depressed with the fear that they will be dependent. There is sudden anxiety, and anxiety about the heart, particularly when stomach conditions are present.

In children the sense of fear is manifest oftentimes in fear of the dark, fear of strangers, fear of imaginary things ; fear that they will not get on in school, timid about going to school, fearful that they will be late to school ; these fears work upon the child life so intensely that they soon wear themselves out and become thoroughly exhausted.

In adults, they find difficulty in concentrating upon their work and their thoughts keep changing about, shifting from one thing to another ; they cannot concentrate because their thoughts get ahead of their work and they become confused. They are not direct thinkers except for a very short time, for the thoughts come so fast that they are entangled by them. This appertains to mental work, but in physical work they have much the same manifestations ; they cannot keep themselves at work steadily ; they cannot " stay put " in one channel for any length of time. They are restless ; they complain that they want to do something but they do not know what it is they want to do. They start tasks they cannot finish, because they tire of them. In their uneasiness, anxiety and restlessness they are compelled to move about, because they cannot keep still. This restlessness is particularly noticeable at the new moon, or if in women, at the approach of the menses.

The change of temperament without any apparent cause is part of the cycle. They become hysterical and go into fits of temper. Young people particularly become hysterical, especially after acute weakening diseases. Psora has fits of anger, yet with these fits of anger there is seldom any desire to harm others in the purely psoric case ; but if the psoric base is united with sycosis or syphilis, there is a decided tendency to harm, or even to kill others.

The greatest force to rouse the evils of the psoric dyscrasia is grief or sorrow. These emotions seem to have particular power in bringing out the exacerbations, and people under the influence of grief and sorrow will often develop immediately some acute sickness.

Psoric patients have much depression of spirits. If the patient is a woman, she will suddenly burst out crying, which relieves the whole condition. When they get into this depressed condition everyone knows of their troubles, because they are not accustomed to silent grief. Melancholy patients on awakening from sleep have heart palpitation, and they become nervous and anxious, with a sense of constriction about the heart ; then they will have flushes of heat. In these conditions they will pass from depression of spirits into moodiness, sulkiness or fits of temper, then suddenly come out of these moods and act like entirely different persons.

The psoric disturbance possesses the very life force, and it is so fundamental in the patient that in order to meet the disturbance a remedy having a marked similarity in the mental traits must be used to overcome the stigma. Psoric manifestations are ameliorated by the eliminative functions, and conditions such as diarrhœa, perspiration, or even a free urination may ameliorate the condition. (In sycotic manifestations we find a general amelioration from eliminations, but not through perspiration, diarrhœa or urination ; sycosis is ameliorated by the unusual eliminations through the mucous surfaces, such as leucorrhœa or free nasal discharges.)

Pathological developments very rarely take place under a purely psoric manifestation. It is only when this taint is united with another stigma that pathological conditions arise ; and when the two (or three) are united in the same individual the vital energy is not powerful enough to overcome the pathological formations. Malignancy is developed in the presence of the combined stigmata, and for that reason these conditions are difficult to treat, and are impossible of real cure under any form of treatment except by stimulating the vital energy. Other conditions difficult of treatment, such as epilepsy and true insanity, are also manifestations of the combined stigmata. These are usually tubercular in their origin, being a grafting of the syphilitic on to the psoric fault.

The vital force or vital energy cannot long endure disturbances to remain latent where more than one stigma is present. Psora seldom if ever develops pathological manifestations when it is alone, and the trouble may remain quiescent, but where there is more than one basic dyscrasia, one is at once inflamed by the other, and disturbances manifest themselves. When one of the latent conditions is psora, it is stirred in all its power, and all that is destructive, hateful and menacing in the psoric stigma will be the first to appear.

In treating the combined stigmata, the most outstanding must be treated first, since we base our method of treatment upon symptom similarity, and where psora is present, psora will be the most outstanding in the symptom totality in the earlier manifestations. This manifestation must be treated first ; then after that is eradicated or considerably lessened, the next most potent dyscrasia, as it expresses itself in the symptomatology, must be treated, until this, too, is eradicated. The treatment should continue in this way, each time treating the most dominant stigma, as expressed by the outward manifestations, until cure is attained.

We are fortunate that many of our most deeply acting remedies have the ability to meet and deal with more than one of these deep underlying conditions ; therefore it is not always necessary, if a remedy be carefully selected, to zigzag a chronic case toward cure. Nevertheless, our treatment must always be based upon the totality of the symptoms as they manifest themselves.

Due to Hahnemann's great discovery of this basic stigma, psora, and his pointing the way in which it can be met, the homœopathic physician has the power to forestall the destructive processes of many chronic diseases and to stop the development of conditions that would inevitably lead to fatal terminations. It is the study of these things and the knowledge of them and of the way to meet them that gives the homœopathic physician the opportunity and the privilege of correcting in childhood and youth these devastating scourges, and developing the future child into his full strength with all of his vital power intact.

CHAPTER XXVI

DISEASE CLASSIFICATION: THE SYPHILITIC STIGMA

THE venereal stigmata (or, as Hahnemann called them, miasms), are fundamentally infections of a specific nature. It is well to bear in mind the *basis* of all infection and of all chronic diseases before we can properly understand the *workings* of a stigmatic disease. Let us consider syphilis, for instance.

This is one of the comparatively modern diseases, and it is the basis for many constitutional troubles. Syphilis is from its inception a constitutional disturbance. Syphilis is supposed to be contracted from an impure coition. Much of the susceptibility and lowering of the defence toward the specific poison is developed and maintained because of the mental attitude of the individual, in that in its very inception it is a violation of his moral standards and therefore reacts upon and lowers the vitality.

Let us consider what happens after an impure coition. Prophylactics seemingly have very little to do with preventing the development of this condition, but there remains a period of about three weeks after the exposure when no symptoms or r ' manifestations of any kind show themselves. This is the period when the disease is taking hold on the system constitutionally, while apparently producing no symptoms. Then the vital energy undertakes to expel the poison by forming a chancre on some part of the body surface, usually the genital organs. In other words, the vital energy is attempting to push out the enemy, and so long as this chancre remains on the surface as an expression of the inward turmoil, no constitutional symptoms appear.

This state may last for months, or even years, provided it is not suppressed. In just the degree that this chancre does not suffer interference does it represent the ability of the vital energy to cope with the intruder. The general treatment among physicians is to cauterize or treat locally this manifestation, such treatment tending to immediately dry the chancre and throw the poison back, by suppression, into the innermost recesses of the system. Then it is that a chain of symptoms begins to develop, showing that the vital energy is profoundly disturbed, and that it is helpless to cope unaided with the enemy.

(Now investigators in the ordinary school of medicine have begun to question whether chancre is not a provision of nature to counteract the syphilitic poison, their theory being that the chancre actually produces within itself antibodies that act defensively against the specific inroads of the disease.)

Usually the next step taken by Nature is to produce an eruption on the body. If this manifestation is in turn treated by suppressive measures, the disease attacks the internal organs, tending always to attack that part of the organism which is least able to resist. It may be the central nervous system ; it may be the arterial system and the heart ; it may be the liver or the intestinal tract. Any or all of the tissues of the body feels the deadening influence of this intruder. These manifestations may be suppressed in one place after another, so that the man lives out his days with this incubus in his system, ever ready to develop into some new manifestation at the most trivial provocation. Grief, sorrow and worry are potent influences to develop these manifestations ; or it may be exposure to the elements, a slight accident, stress of business relationship, or any one of many other causes, that starts the irritation ; but unless this is met by the art of the similar antisyphilitic remedy, he passes his days in discomfort and distress and comes to a premature old age.

This stigma has its effect upon the protozoon, and the offspring shows the effect in many ways. When the offspring is affected with the syphilitic taint he will not show the direct effect in the primary chancre or ulcer, for by the time the disease has passed into the second generation the fault has become thoroughly married to the life forces and it becomes a part of his being. This results in many constitutional tendencies such as deformities, chronic catarrhal conditions of the nose and throat, malformations of the teeth and of the bony structure, ulcers and many other manifestations. In the second generation we find none of the primary local manifestations, for the manifestations have changed their character, showing that the economy is thoroughly impregnated with the deadening and destructive effect of the stigma.

In the primary disturbance we may find that this infection of syphilis becomes grafted on to a psoric base. Here we have a complication of troubles, and just as each of these stigmata is a problem in itself, the union of the two becomes a much more complicated problem, requiring great patience and skill to solve. Usually in this union of psora and syphilis the psoric symptoms predominate, and here the predominant symptoms of psora must be treated first with the antipsoric *simillimum*, for the syphilis is largely hidden, and we must strive to help the vital force to throw off the greater and more predominant incubus which the patient manifests.

After the patient responds to the remedy by a decided improvement in the conditions first prescribed for, and the psoric condition is largely obliterated, we must change our tactics, for then the syphilitic dyscrasia will show itself and become prominent. Then the symptoms must be met with the antisyphilitic *simillimum*, or the remedy that is most similar and adapted to syphilitic symptoms, to which we will be guided by the similitude of the remedy.

The patient who is suffering from syphilis in a latent state or who manifests the inherited stigma presents a picture that is very easy to recognize ; and this is probably the easiest of the miasms, or stigmata, to treat. Patients with inherited or latent syphilis are mentally dull, heavy, stupid and especially stubborn, sullen, morose, and usually suspicious. They are always depressed, but in the depression they keep their troubles to themselves and sulk over them. These are the people who develop fixed ideas, which are not eradicated by any amount of explanation or talk. Their mental powers are slow in reaction ; they become melancholy, and condemn themselves. They like to be alone, yet desire to escape from themselves as well as from others. In their slowness of comprehension the thoughts they had in starting a sentence will vanish, they forget what they were about to say, and they find it hard to get back into the track of their conversation. If they are reading, they read a few lines, and then they must re-read it to comprehend it.

They are always worse at night ; all the symptoms develop more after the sun goes down. There is oppression, restlessness and anxiety at night ; they dread the night because it is so oppressive. Restlessness is so great that it drives them out of bed.

We must remember that the tubercular patient is manifesting the union of the syphilitic and the psoric dyscrasias. Oftentimes we find the child who has inherited this stigmatic combination has a tendency toward tuberculosis ; this child presents the picture of the " problem child " in the school, being slow of comprehension, dull, unable to keep a line of thought ; he is unsocial, keeps to himself and becomes morose and sullen. No greater service can be rendered to society than to meet these conditions of the problem child of school age and under, with the homœopathic treatment, using as weapons the antisyphilitic and antipsoric remedies as they are indicated. This is the only treatment that will put these children into the sphere where they will be able to develop normally and become useful, happy citizens.

In patients manifesting the syphilitic stigma, if we are so fortunate as to observe the appearance of external manifestations or unusual discharges we will observe also that the patient is greatly improved in general and his mental state will seemingly become more normal. This is true if a catarrhal or leucorrhœal discharge is established ; it is true if an old ulcer, perhaps of the leg, opens up and discharges ; and so long as these avenues of escape are active the patient will be more normal. However, the natural avenues of elimination do not ameliorate the patient ; sweating aggravates rather than ameliorates, and natural sweat, profuse urination and diarrhœas never ameliorate the syphilitic conditions, except in constitutions such as the tubercular, which are a combination of the syphilitic and the psoric, and this is due to the general amelioration of all psoric manifestations from these natural avenues of elimination. In tubercular children a hæmorrhage from the nose will clear up the mental state for some time ; and in tubercular adults nosebleeds will clear up old neuralgias.

Now the degenerates and criminals and criminally insane are either sycotic or syphilitic in their stigmatic inheritances. Many of the criminally insane and degenerates could be very greatly benefited and probably cured by some of the anti-syphilitic remedies.

Let us take up some of the symptoms of the head as manifest in the syphilitic patient. These headaches usually come on in the night and are almost always in the back of the head ; they will ache all night, get better in the morning, only to come on again at night. The headaches are dull, heavy, yet lancinating ; they are persistently constant at the base of the brain or on one side.

The headaches that come on Sundays or when they are away from their usual vocations are usually psoric and syphilitic combinations. Syphilitic headaches are usually < riding, > by motion, < by exertion, either mental or physical. They are usually accompanied by a great deal of coldness of the body, sadness and prostration. They are < by warmth or heat and > by cold applications ; < by quiet rest, by lying down at night and by sleep, and > by nose-bleed. (Note the indications for the syphilitic headache as being almost exactly opposite those of the psoric type, which are > by rest, by lying down, > by hot applications ; the psoric headaches come on in the daytime while the syphilitic are manifest at night.)

Oftentimes the syphilitic patient complains of a band about the head, which is probably due to a slight effusion from the meningeal surfaces. A child with these syphilitic headaches will bore his head into the pillow or roll the head from side to side. Without the antisyphilitic remedy these headaches are not easily amenable to treatment. Some people complain that before these headaches they experience a ravenous hunger ; these manifestations are a combination of syphilis and psora.

The syphilitic stigma shows many types of vertigo, but especially those at the base of the brain. These may be present also in the sycotic stigma, but they are especially apt to be present in the tubercular diathesis, the combination of syphilis and psora. Since both syphilis and psora have marked vertigo, the union of the two stresses this symptom in a marked degree.

The symptom of high blood pressure is caused, from the structural point of view, by a thickening of the arterial coats or an attack of nephritic obstruction, and is an expression of an actual change of structure in the arterial system. Change of structure does not occur in uncomplicated psora, but when the psoric dyscrasia is combined with the syphilitic, structural changes do take place, and in this manifestation we have an expression of the combination of the two stigmata.

The appearance of people suffering from the syphilitic stigma often tells the story at a glance, for we observe that the head is large and bulging, the hair is moist, gluey, greasy, and with an offensive odour ; the hair falls out in bunches, beginning first on the vertex and then on the temples. The hair on the eyebrows and eyelashes falls, and the hair in the beard falls. The hairs in the beard are often ingrowing, and suppurate ; elderly people often complain that the hairs in the eyelashes break and turn inward, causing much irritation in the conjunctiva.

Closer examination shows that in these greatly enlarged heads the sutures are soft ; the fontanelles remain open after the normal time of closing, and there is a general hydrocephaloid appearance of the head.

The scalp is moist in general. The scalp perspires and the hair becomes wet ; the scalp perspires when they are asleep or when they are awake. The eruptions on the scalp are almost always moist, with thick yellow crusts, from under which thick yellow pus oozes. The eczemas about and behind the ears having thick fœtid pus, and the cracks about the ear and in the aural canal, are a grafting of the syphilitic stigma on to the psoric. In the tubercular patient the eruptions on the scalp are < by bathing.

The eyes are astigmatic, and this syphilitic dyscrasia has deformities of the lens and of the cornea, and all refractory changes are related to this stigma. Remember that syphilis deforms everything ; psora alone and by itself never causes deformities, but in the combination of the two we find a great many deformities.

Ulceration is the mark of the syphilitic. You will find in these patients ulcerations of the cornea ; ulcerations of the lids. A peculiar reaction of these patients is that they are intolerant of artificial light. You will hear them say that they cannot read or work by artificial light. This corresponds with the period of aggravation of the syphilitic miasm.

Ptosis of the lids and the neuralgias of the eyes and the head come under the syphilitic group. These neuralgias are < at night and < from heat.

Discharges from the eyes in these conditions are greenish or greenish-yellow in colour. This is present also in sycotic people, or in people with tubercular troubles. Granulations of the lids, as well as styes, are of the tubercular type.

In babes and children and young people under twenty years of age you often find very widely dilated pupils ; this is an indication of the tubercular diathesis.

In tubercularly inclined children you find structural changes in the ear. Everything that attacks them, such as colds or sore throats or any of the so-called acute diseases, shows its relationship to the stigmatic combination by suppurations of the ear. This suppuration, no matter how painful it may be, is the safety-valve of child life. In all of these ear manifestations, the tendency to the night aggravation is very marked ; they will be all right during the day, but from sun-down to sun-up the characteristic aggravation shows itself. In every eruptive disease there is an accompaniment of middle ear trouble in these children, and they will continue this process until the antipsoric and anti-syphilitic remedies have done their beneficial work.

Very often in these stigmatic complications of the ear there is more or less discharge, and so long as the discharge from the ear continues the patient improves in general health. Sometimes this discharge from the ear will continue for years, and the health will remain fairly good. However, if the discharge is suppressed, the patient's health suffers greatly.

In appearance, these patients develop very large ears. The lobe of the ear is pale, white and transparent

In the syphilitic dyscrasia the sense of smell is lost, and the nose bleeds very readily, especially when there is the complication with psora, in the pre-tubercular stage. The pre-tubercular child will have hæmorrhages from the nose at the slightest provocation. At the same time they are subject to severe headaches, but the hæmorrhages relieve the head symptoms.

Acne indurata of the nose depends upon the union of the psoric and the syphilitic conditions. By many this condition is considered impossible of cure, yet with the knowledge of its stigmatic origin it may be removed and the patient brought to a better state of health.

One of the cardinal signs of the syphilitic taint is the destruction of tissue. This is the only stigma in which the bones of the nose are destroyed. Infants and children who have " snuffles " are manifesting either the syphilitic or sycotic taint. The syphilitic expression in the nose is by many scabs and crusts, which are dark greenish to brown or black. These are not always offensive in odour, but in the tubercular diathesis these manifestations have the odour of old cheese, and there is a thick yellow discharge that drops back into the throat.

In the hay fever type of troubles, which is one of the most troublesome conditions we have to deal with, we have as a base the psoric, the syphilitic and the sycotic. The sycotic remains latent during the active period, but will come out later, after proper treatment has been instituted. These cases are always difficult to treat, and still more difficult when serum or vaccine treatment has been given.

In the tubercular diathesis, there are circumscribed red spots on the cheeks of adults or children, before any other manifestations show themselves ; there are also hot flushes other than at the climacteric period. The characteristic appearance of the syphilitic stigma is a greyish, greasy face. There are deep fissures, especially in the lips ; swelling and œdema of the face in the pre-tubercular patients, in the morning after waking and after a nap. Moles may be a manifestation of either the syphilitic or sycotic stigma.

In the fevers of the tubercular patient the face is pale, with circumscribed redness on the cheekbones : in the morning the face is intensely pale. The children with ashy grey faces and the appearance of marasmus are basically syphilitic. The syphilitic stigma destroys not only the tissues, but it destroys also the power of the body to assimilate the proper materials from food. On the other hand, the tubercular child may be plump, with a white, clear skin and long, beautiful silky eyelashes. In these children the face and head and about the back of the neck perspire freely.

In the mouth we find the characteristic tell-tale of the syphilitic taint, even though the child may appear well otherwise. Pathological and structural changes take place in the dental arch and the teeth come through deformed, irregular in shape and irregular in order of eruption. The teeth often decay before they are entirely through the gums.

These little patients get sick every time a tooth comes, and they are constantly having trouble with one thing after another ; persistently taking cold ; persistently having upset stomachs ; exceedingly susceptible to any change in the weather. They have very flabby muscles and they develop large cervical glands. The adenoid tissue is always involved and the enlarged tonsils are a prominent manifestation.

Actual ulcers occur in the mouth. Psora never develops ulcers of itself, but the syphilitic taint is very prone to this manifestation. In the tubercular type there is a putrid, sweet taste in the mouth ; more of a metallic taste in the purely syphilitic dyscrasia ; in the union of syphilis and psora we find a saliva that is ropy and viscid with a bloody taste.

The tubercular type of patients have ravenous hunger ; hunger immediately after a full meal ; hunger at all times ; there is no time they cannot eat. There is much craving for unaccountable things, like the craving for acids, for sweets ; a longing to chew chalk, lime and pencils ; a craving for indigestible things. The craving for salt is particularly noticeable in the tubercular diathesis. It will be noted that here also the psoric influence is strong, in that psora has many cravings, and great hunger.

In these unnatural cravings we have the key to assist many people whom we may consider to lack temperance in eating and drinking. They are particularly prone to crave spirituous liquors and it is the tubercular diathesis which produces the people who are apt to become drunkards, for you must remember that these are the people who bear about with them the combined power of psora and syphilis. By looking well to our indications we can give these people a great deal of help to overcome these unnatural cravings, and at the same time gradually eliminate the stigma.

Chapter XXVII

DISEASE CLASSIFICATION : THE SYPHILITIC STIGMA, continued

It has been said that the patient afflicted with the syphilitic taint suffers from structural changes ; yet the emotional sphere in the purely syphilitic patient is not seriously affected. For this reason, in the syphilitic patient we find less subjective symptoms ; there is little of the supersensitiveness, and less desires, cravings and longings than in the psoric patient. The syphilitic patient actually suffers much less than the psoric ; the mental sphere has not been so much invaded, for the syphilitic stigma is not so thoroughly established through untold centuries of time as the psoric, and because it is not so thoroughly a part of the very essence of man's spirit we have a far better chance to eradicate the dyscrasia.

The very earmarks of the various stigmata show their respective characters. The psoric itches, and appears unclean, unwashed. The syphilitic ulcerates and the bony structure is changed. The sycotic infiltrates and is corroded by its discharges.

Psora is the stigma which shows little on the side of objective symptoms, but expresses itself through the mental and emotional reactions. For this reason the patient of a tubercular diathesis reflects many subjective symptoms in comparison with the purely syphilitic for, as has been pointed out before, the tubercular is the combination of the psoric and syphilitic. In this combination we find all the mental and emotional reactions, the subjective symptoms, of the predominant parent, psora, and the pathological and destructive changes of the younger parent, syphilis.

Syphilis alone has few cravings in the way of food ; it is averse to meats, but aside from that negative symptom there is little that we note in the way of appetite. Compare that state with the tubercular cravings, which were pointed out in the last chapter.

The frequent, unsatisfied hunger ; the craving for meat and potatoes when nothing else will satisfy ; the craving for salt ; craving for indigestible things ; the inability to assimilate much starch ; these marked symptoms of appetite show the psoric parentage of the tubercular diathesis.

In the syphilitic-psoric type we find the changes in the chest wall, which are structural changes in the bone contours. The chest wall is narrow and may be more shallow than normal ; even the action of the diaphragm is limited. While there may be no structural changes in the lung itself, there is less air capacity and less residual air in the lung. The very structural changes eventually bring about occlusion of the air cells and the formation of foci, for these people are very poor breathers ; the pumping power is so cramped that they are incapable of supplying sufficient oxygen for the body needs. This is shown in the anæmic and chlorotic conditions, as well as in the tubercular. The tuberculosis produces its destruction by first cramping the aeration of the red blood cell through the formation of the bony structure. Because breathing is a difficult process they become averse to fresh air, and will survive for a long time in a close, breathed-over atmosphere.

Long before tuberculosis develops, sometimes even years before, you may notice a symptom of the latent diathesis : on the least exposure to cold the patient develops a deep, hoarse cough. This will be repeated many, many times before there is actual development of the tuberculosis. The purely syphilitic patient has a short, barking cough ; this is sometimes true of the early tubercular stages.

The tubercular expectoration is purulent, greenish-yellow, often offensive ; usually sweetish or salty to his taste. We can usually depend upon the salty or sweetish taste as being a characteristic of this dyscrasia.

There is the everlastingly tired feeling of the tubercular type ; (the psoric is always ready to lie down) ; the tubercular patient is better in the daytime and worse as night comes on, showing the syphilitic influence. The syphilitic patients should be sun-worshippers in type, for they are always better during the daylight hours, and all conditions are < at night. The tubercular people suffer from neuralgias, prosopalgias, sciaticas, insomnias, hysterias, and all the nervous symptoms peculiar to the diathesis. They may have for years persistent headaches ; this may precede the actual tubercular development. Hysterical and other nervous symptoms often precede the tubercular manifestation, and when the lung condition improves the hysteria will return ; when the hysteria improves the lung condition takes on renewed activity. Often a severe dysmenorrhœa will stay for a time the disease progress in the lung itself. In other words, the pre-tubercular manifestations are more psoric than syphilitic ; but the structure predisposing to develop the lung condition is syphilitic.

When children cry out in their sleep we may take this to be an indication of the tubercular diathesis, which may take on a meningeal form when it develops. Look carefully to all night aggravations, especially in children, to see if they are not pre-tubercular indications.

The tubercular diathesis has many heart symptoms, showing the psoric parentage. There is much palpitation. In the psoric this is due to uterine or gastric irritations and disturbances ; in the sycotic patients the heart manifestations are reflexes of rheumatic conditions. In the syphilitic and sycotic stigmata we find little mental disturbance accompanying the heart conditions, even when the conditions are critical ; it is the psoric patient who worries about his heart condition and rarely succumbs to it. It is the syphilitic or sycotic patient who may have for years a slight dyspnœa and occasionally slight pains, or perhaps no symptoms at all, but they die suddenly and without warning.

In the tubercular, as in the psoric heart conditions, the patients want to keep still ; they are much < by higher altitudes; cannot climb stairs or ascend hills; cannot breathe well on ascending; have not the proper amount of room for air. They have no difficulty in descending. With this heart condition there is a cyanosis that is often painful. There is a gradual falling away in flesh in these conditions. The syphilitic dropsies and anasarcas are greater than the sycotic.

Lymphatic involvement of the abdomen is of tubercular origin, as are the hernias ; the muscles lack tone.

Hereditary syphilitic troubles in children sometimes produce a very watery discharge that almost completely drains the system of its vital fluids and unless promptly corrected death ensues. The cholera infantum types of diarrhœa are syphilitic ; we often find tubercular diarrhœas which simulate the cholera infantum, but they do not as rapidly drain the system. In the tubercular diarrhœas we find the < in the night or the early morning, driving the patient out of bed, and < by cold, showing the syphilitic relationship. The tubercular child often cannot assimilate cows' milk in any form ; the casein has to be modified before it can be digested at all. These are the children who have undigested curds in the loose stool.

There is a close relationship between the ability to take the lime salts from food and these diarrhœas of tubercular children ; this is the reason for the difficult and irregular dentition and the craving for the elements which the body needs ; they cannot assimilate the necessary elements from their food. The diarrhœas of the syphilitic child who is strongly tainted with sycosis will probably call for some such remedy as *Croton tig.* or *Sarsaparilla.*

The tubercular stool is apt to be slimy, bloody, with a musty, mouldy smell ; nausea and gagging before stools and prostration with a desire to be left alone after stools. Hæmorrhages from the rectum are signposts of tuberculosis, although there are bleeding hæmorrhoids in sycosis. Tubercular patients are troubled with pin worms and seat worms. The characteristic alternation of symptoms in the tubercular patient may be noted in the alternation of rectal diseases with heart, chest or lung troubles, especially in asthma or respiratory difficulties. Very often, operated or suppressed hæmorrhoids will be followed by asthmatic manifestations, often accompanied by heart troubles.

In the rectum, strictures, sinuses, fistulas and pockets are all of tubercular origin, but these conditions are much more frequent and in much aggravated form when combined with the sycotic stigma. Cancerous manifestations of the rectum are a combination of the tubercular and sycotic ; in other words, they are a manifestation of the combined destructive force of the three stigmata. Psora alone never reaches to pathological changes; yet without the psoric element malignancies will never develop.

In the urinary tract all of the stigmata may manifest themselves, but most frequently these manifestations are psoric and sycotic; here also the combined assault of all three stigmata are represented in the malignancies. The diabetic patient is as a rule strongly tubercular; sometimes in these conditions there is a strong taint of the sycotic, which makes the condition much more malignant. We never see marked tissue changes or fibrous growths without the presence of the three stigmata, although the tubercular and sycotic are represented in the majority of cases of Bright's disease. While the psoric element is present in these conditions, it is not in as marked degree as the syphilitic and sycotic.

Nocturnal enuresis, with the < during sleep and soon after falling asleep, are tubercular; and nightly emissions also are a combination of the syphilitic and psoric taints. Usually prostatic troubles may be classed under the union of these two stigmata.

Syphilis seldom attacks the ovaries or the uterus. In pathological conditions we occasionally find a manifestation of the tubercular diathesis, but this is because of the psoric affinity for functional and emotional disturbances and not because of the syphilitic influence toward these organs.

The syphilitic stigma attacks the long bones; the growing pains of children are syphilitic, especially when < at night, < in storms or on change of weather. This stigma causes destruction of tissue partly because it hampers assimilation of the necessary elements, and we see the result in rickets of children; they cannot assimilate from their food what they require to make the bones sufficiently hard to support their weight without bending.

The nails of these patients are characteristic, being paper-thin, spoon-shaped and bending and tearing easily. Where the nails are irregular, brittle, break and split easily, and with many hangnails, this is an unfailing sign of the tubercular; these nails are also spotted, or with white specks, and scalloped edges. Felons about the nail are a manifestation of the combined effects of syphilis and psora, as are all periosteal affections.

The psoric-syphilitic patients cannot endure much cold, yet they cannot endure much heat ; the heat from the stove may drive them from the room.

Chilblains are a combination of all the stigmata. Anyone who has endured the torments of this affliction can readily understand how willing these sufferers are to accept any form of treatment which promises some relief ; yet a suppression of this manifestation brings in its train a succession of all sorts of nervous diseases and many other serious conditions, even to malignancies.

Corns and like hypertrophies are tubercular manifestations. Boils are usually psoric, but when there is much suppuration and pain it is usually a combination of the psoric and syphilitic manifestations. It is characteristic of psoric eruptions that they tend to dry down and scale off rather than to suppurate. However, the appearance of boils after the administration of the antipsoric remedy is a welcome and encouraging indication.

Children who have weak wrist and ankle joints, who have difficulty in holding on to objects, who drop things easily, who are clumsy in getting about and stumble over a straw, are manifesting the effects of the combined syphilis and psora, for this combination affects the tendons about the joints by weakening them so that they will not stand the strain of much use.

As we naturally expect, there are a great many skin manifestations with the syphilitic miasm and in the tubercular dyscrasia. There are pustular eruptions which suppurate, and eruptions occur especially about the joints or in the flexures of the body. These eruptions are quite prone to arrange themselves in crescentic formation. In colour they are coppery or brownish, but sometimes very red at the base of the pustules. The most striking characteristic of these syphilitic eruptions is that they do not itch, and there is very little soreness. If these eruptions progress to scaling and crusts, as they usually do, these are very thick and occur in patches or circumscribed spots.

The gangrenes of the skin and dry gangrenes show the destructiveness of the syphilitic stigma.

Skin affections with glandular involvement are frequent.

Occasionally psoriasis shows itself. Psoriasis has been called the marriage of all the miasms, or stigmata, but its characteristics are predominantly psoric and sycotic. Another type of eruption where all the stigmata are present is the fishscale eruption. In this condition we have the dryness of psora, the squamous character of the syphilitic eruption and the moles and warts of sycosis.

Varicose veins are of tubercular origin. Varicose ulcers are the last destructive manifestation on the skin of the syphilitic taint. In this stigma, too, we see the ecchymoses and hæmorrhagic conditions into the skin ; purpureal conditions are all manifestations of the syphilitic taint.

Erysipelatous and carcinomatous conditions, epithelioma and lupus, are all manifestations of the union of the three stigmata. In acute exanthematous diseases we see the tubercular diathesis. These conditions show the psora in the severity of the attack, but the profound prostration from the lowered vitality is the mark of the syphilitic taint. Urticarias occur in the tubercular diathesis. Marked freckling is also a manifestation of the tubercular diathesis ; this has the clear, almost transparent skin of the tubercular patient, with the pigmentation of the psoric. Impetigo will readily develop in the combination of the psoric and syphilitic stigmata, while those without this dyscrasia will not become infected.

We often find patients with slight wounds that heal very slowly or not at all ; this condition is due to the union of the syphilitic and psoric influences. In this same category we may place the stitch abscesses which occur following operative measures, in hospitals and under the best of sanitary conditions.

We have spoken a great deal of the tubercular diathesis as being a combination of the syphilitic and psoric stigmata. The scrofulous diathesis is also a combination of these two stigmata, but it differs in the proportionate degree of the presence of the taints, and is further influenced by the suppressive measures of crude drugging. Probably environment and circumstances have some bearing on it also. However, the suppression is a strong factor in its individual expression, because this has buried it deeper in the system.

The scrofulous diathesis manifests itself largely by the involvement of the glandular system, particularly the lymphatics. While many authorities have classed scrofula as psoric, its relation may be traced by its manifestations. Psora has no glandular involvement, but syphilis has a particular affinity for glandular tissue. Scrofula has many symptoms in common with psora, but it has the same tendency to ulceration as syphilis ; this relationship may be seen also in the purulent discharges and decomposition of the exudations. Scrofula has the same tendency as syphilis to locate in the organs of the special senses, such as the eyes, ears, nose, lips, etc. The pernicious anæmia of the scrofulous patient resembles very closely the syphilitic parent, and shows its kinship to the tubercular diathesis.

Chapter XXVIII

SYPHILIS

WE have spoken of the psoric miasm as being closely related to the deficiency diseases, so called. Now on the same basis of the table of atomic weights in relation to disease conditions we are considering the problem of the venereal taints, syphilis and sycosis. Just as we find the remedies pre-eminently antipsoric in the lower register of atomic weights—below 53—and just as we find these closely related to the constructive elements in living tissue, so we find the elements with the highest powers of destruction in the upper and highest registers of atomic weights.

It is to be remembered that the constructive elements are, as Millikan states, "in their state of maximum stability already; they have no energy to give up in the disintegrating process. They can only be broken apart by working upon them, or by supplying energy to them. . . .". However, when we consider the radioactive elements we find the problem an entirely different one, and necessarily their homœopathic field of action will be different. We cannot expect construction from essentially destructive forces, so long as they remain in their natural state.

Millikan tells us that the process of radioactive disintegration is a process that can take place only in the case of a very few of the very heavy elements; that radioactivity is a heat-evolving (exothermic) process; that it is self-destructive in that it gives off of itself in the process and after this process has continued a sufficient length of time the original substance is itself changed; it has become more inert and has less and less radioactive properties and powers. We are told that Uranium, after it has discharged its alpha particles for a considerable period of time (geologically considered) has become so much lighter in atomic weight that we recognize it as Thorium; this eventually is worn down into Radium, and this in turn disintegrates into Lead.

|F - 15ᴇ

Thus we see that these radioactive elements have no choice; they cannot rest in their ceaseless self-destruction, and they cannot come in contact with other substances without in turn destroying them.

We have stated that syphilis is the only miasm or stigma that actually destroys living tissue. It destroys not only soft tissues but bony tissues, and attacks the very life of the unborn child. If, after repeated abortions, a child is born to a parent having this marked taint, we frequently find the tissues so disturbed by the attack of the disease that it were better the child had died. If the child is not actually disfigured, and attains the age of puberty, we are sure to find this cruel stamp upon it. The symptoms of this miasm as they appear all down its trail have been stated in detail previously. Now we have to consider the chemical affinity of certain elements to the disease taint—in other words, the foreordained homœopathicity.

If Sulphur is the remedy that most clearly typifies the psoric classification, so Mercury is the closest remedial synonym for the syphilitic. We find Mercury in the higher range of elements; in fact, from Osmium (76) onward we may consider the proven range of the antisyphilitics. Reference to the homœopathic materia medica will give us a clear outline of the symptomatology of Osmium, Iridium, Platinum, Aurum, Mercury, Plumbum, Bismuth, Radium and Uranium. We have not sufficient provings of some of the other elements in this range. But we often find some of the remedies indicated in these conditions that come in the lower, or constructive, register. How are we to account for this?

McMillan, Thornton and Lawrence of the University of California reported before the National Academy of Sciences in 1935 that they had developed a process whereby certain of the lower elements had been made radioactive. This end was accomplished by " breaking through the enormously high energy barrier that surrounds the nucleus of the atom " and for this purpose they employed a special apparatus, perfected for the purpose, with a very low amperage and very high voltage. Copper and sodium chloride were both made artificially radioactive, and the sodium chloride remains radioactive in solution, even when injected into the tissues.

They were quoted as stating further : " A single drop of water contains enough energy to supply 200 horse power continuously for a year, but at present it takes more energy to break into the atom than is released. When this ratio can be reversed atomic energy will be available."

Millikan says of the more common and lighter elements (such as sodium, for instance) : " Man can probably learn to disintegrate them, but he will always do it ' by the sweat of his brow.' "

Here again we see that radioactivity and disintegration are a common thought, and this applies equally to the syphilitic stigma.

We frequently find a patient susceptible to the action of *Natrum mur.* in potentiated form—that is, the form in which the energies have been released by applied force in the form of succussion—who has partaken repeatedly and frequently of salt in the diet with no appreciable vital effect. Yet in the continued attack by force and motion upon the construction of the sodium atom, these energies have been released so that the substance is changed in its very essentials, and it takes on and retains an artificial radioactivity which activates it for a considerable period of time. So it is with many other substances, seemingly inert in their natural state, which take on activity under the homœopathic potentiation.

CHAPTER **XXIX**

DISEASE CLASSIFICATION : SYCOSIS

SYCOSIS is generally understood to be the gonorrhœal poison. We should make the distinction clear between gonorrhœa and sycosis. Gonorrhœa is the acute infection of the gonococci, which takes from five to ten days to develop a urethritis after an exposure. During this incubation period it is purely an infection ; then the local manifestations are thrown outward by Nature at the point of attack as a resentment of the vital energy to the infection. If the gonorrhœa is thoroughly and completely cured, practically no sycosis ever develops. Sycosis is established after a suppressed gonorrhœa, when the acute infection is driven in upon the vital energy by external methods of suppression, and it then becomes a systematic stigma, permeating every living cell of the organism, and transmitting its deadly destructive forces to the offspring as well as retaining the full destructiveness of its power in the original individual, and impregnating the mother of the child.

The suppressed gonorrhœal infection is very apt to first show itself in attacking the blood and producing an anæmic condition, and a general catarrhal condition is set up. Oftentimes an inflammatory rheumatism develops ; inflammation follows in the soft tissues, and changes in the fibre of the muscles. In fact, the whole organism becomes involved. Sometimes a stasis develops in the lymphatics ; there is a swelling in the groin following the suppression, and inflammation in the prostatic gland.

These are the symptoms that are first produced after a suppression, showing that the whole organism is involved and in the grip of this destructive force. Seldom do we get these constitutional symptoms when the initial gonorrhœa is cured by the homœopathically indicated remedy, and if there is any constitutional taint, it is in a mild form.

The transmission of this gonorrhœal poison, or sycotic poison, as the case may be, is transmitted in the stage into which the infecting individual has arrived. If it is a true gonorrhœal infection, true gonorrhœa will be transmitted ; but if it has reached the secondary stage (which usually comes on three months after the first stage has subsided, and may be delayed a full year) the contracting party will develop the condition at the same stage as the infector.

The secondary and tertiary symptoms of sycosis can be entirely eradicated by homœopathic treatment.

In the secondary period of sycosis almost every disease that may arise takes on an inflammatory nature in some form ; it may be acute, subacute or chronic, and it may vary from very mild to very malignant fevers.

We know how frequently we see cases where soon after marriage a perfectly healthy, robust girl begins to droop and becomes ill. This is because the secondary symptoms of sycosis have been transmitted to the extensive mucous surfaces of the female organs. Oftentimes it is a single organ that becomes involved, like the ovary with its cystic manifestations, or a fallopian tube manifests inflammation ; again they may show a very anæmic state of the blood, and when this anæmic condition arises it affects every part of her organism, coming on gradually, slowly, until her whole system is permeated. She becomes pallid, drawn, puffy ; there is no stamina to the muscles. The anæmic condition arises from this stigma because sycosis destroys the red blood cells through imperfect oxidization of food.

This may be a forerunner of carcinomatous conditions of the breast or uterus ; diabetes, Bright's disease, or numerous other diseases of this type, largely dependent upon previously existing taints in her own system. Sycotic manifestations are characterized by slowness of recovery ; the subject is constantly slipping backward because of the destructive character of the stigma, whenever he gets an acute manifestation.

The sycotic patient is exceedingly suspicious. The suspicion extends to the point where he dare not trust himself, and he must go back and repeat what he has done or said, and wonders if he has said just what he means ; he

goes back and starts again. He is suspicious that he will
be misunderstood, that his hearers will give the wrong
meaning to what he is attempting to convey. This suspicion,
when turned upon others, leads to the worst forms of jealousy
of his friends, for he knows full well that he is not understood.
The sycotic taint develops the worst forms of degeneracy
because of the basic suspicion and jealousy, patients will
resort to any and all means of vindicating themselves in
their own light. This is the most markedly degenerate of the
stigmata, in its suspicion, its quarrelsomeness, its tendency
to harm others and to harm animals. This produces the
worst forms of cruelty and cunning deceit and the worst
forms of mania of any of the stigmata.

The sycotic patient is cross and irritable ; he is absent-
minded in certain things, and finds difficulty in getting the
right word ; the more he looks at the word after he has
written it, the more strange it seems and the less confident
he is that it is right. He forgets recent happenings, but
remembers distant events very clearly. Sycosis, like the
syphilitic stigma, has the mark of self-condemnation, which
is the moral reaction to the inception of the disease state.

Here, too, we find the fixed ideas, as in syphilis, and in
the union of the two stigmata these characteristics are much
more marked ; there is also the same slow mental power.
The sycotic is disposed to fits of anger, and when the syphilitic
taint is also present these people present the picture of the
sullen, smouldering type that threaten to break out into
dangerous manifestations. Sycosis, coupled with psora, is
the basis of most criminal insanity and of most suicides ;
degenerates are sycotic or syphilitic, or result from the
combined destructiveness of the two stigmata.

When some external manifestation occurs, such as a
catarrhal condition, a leucorrhœa, or even the return of the
menstrual period, there is a general amelioration of the
mental condition. The mental condition may be much >
when warts or fibrous growths appear; they are always > in
general from the return or breaking open of old ulcers or old
sores, and markedly > by the return of acute gonorrhœal
manifestations. Pains often alternate with the leucorrhœa.
While there is much amelioration by eliminative processes,

natural eliminations, such as diarrhœa, free urination, or even perspiration, does not ameliorate.

All the miasms, or stigmata, have many head symptoms. The headache in the vertex is sycotic in its origin ; or there may be frontal headache. These are < lying down and at night, especially < after midnight. There are feverish headaches of children. This patient is restless and wants to be kept in motion, which >. The head symptoms resemble the syphilitic in that they have the night aggravations, and there is the same type of vertigo at the base of the brain.

The hair falls out in circular spots ; the hair of the beard falls. The sycotic scalp perspires, but there are not the moist, matting eruptions of syphilis.

Sycosis never gives a true ulcer ; the sycotic manifestations are more overgrowth of tissue than destructive of tissue. There are many warts and warty growths ; these are sycotic signposts. Moles and papillomata may be either syphilitic or sycotic. Deposits of gouty concretions characterize this stigma.

Arthritic troubles of the eye are a combination of sycosis and psora ; there are also neuralgias which are < on change of weather, < change of barometer, < rainy weather.

The sycotic usually has a red nose with prominent capillaries. The sense of smell is lost. Children with "snuffles" are usually syphilitic or sycotic ; the sycotic stigma has moist snuffles, but without ulcerations or crusts ; the discharge is purulent, scanty, with the odour of fishbrine.

The fishbrine odour is characteristic of the sycotic taint, and it may appear in all the discharges, but especially in the discharges from the genital tract. The sycotic discharges, like the tubercular, are greenish or greenish-yellow.

There is often nasal stoppage due to thickening of the membranes and to enlargement of the turbinated bones. Except in acute colds the discharges are scanty. The slightest amount of discharge, however, > the patient.

Hay fever conditions, which are exceedingly difficult of cure under ordinary treatment, are more easily understood when we remember that they are an expression of syphilis and latent sycosis, very often with a psoric taint. Erysipelas is a combination of the psoric and sycotic stigmata.

The sycotic patient is especially liable to rheumatic troubles, and where this taint appears, especially if there has been any attempt at suppression of the rheumatic manifestations, we find reflex troubles in the heart, with violent hammering and beating.

In the combination of sycosis and psora we get the right soil for valvular and cardiac disturbances with changes in the organic structure ; these are the conditions that cause the fatalities. With these sycotic heart conditions there is none of the fear and apprehension that we find in the psoric patient. The syphilitic and sycotic heart conditions are much more dangerous than the psoric, but the psoric patient worries about his condition, takes his pulse frequently, fears death and remains quiet, while the syphilitic and sycotic patients have no mental distress, and may have no subjective heart symptoms ; but they die suddenly and without warning.

If there are pains about the heart and dyspnœa, these conditions are > from gentle exercise, as slow walking or riding. When there is any trouble about the heart in sycotic patients there is usually some dyspnœa. When the heart condition is of rheumatic origin, however, there is sometimes severe pain, very much < by motion. These patients have a soft, slow, easily compressible pulse ; the valves are roughened, the muscles become flabby and soft, and in long-continued cases they lack power. As a rule these patients are fleshy and puffy ; their obesity is the cause of their dyspnœa.

Frequently the face becomes bluish and cyanotic, sometimes with venous congestion. The cyanotic condition in these patients is not painful. The anasarcas never become very extensive, because these patients die before the anasarca has time to manifest itself to any degree ; they snuff out like a candle. These conditions are very much < by high living, rich spicy food or spirituous liquors.

Meats arouse the latent sycosis as in psora. The sycotic patient should take meat sparingly, and it is better for him to use more freely of nuts, beans or cheese. Gouty conditions cannot digest meats. He craves beer, and while this

is not a desirable element of his diet, it causes much less <
than do wines.

He is usually < by eating any food, and > by lying on
the stomach or by pressure.

His taste is musty or fishy. His pains are always colicky
in nature, especially in the abdomen, and they are > by
bending double and by hard pressure. In fact, we hear of
his colic so frequently that we get tired of the story. There
are occasional diarrhœas, but always preceded and accompanied by the colic, griping and tenesmus. The stools are
gushing and ejaculated forcibly. The colic and stools of
Rheum., Cham. and *Mag. carb.* are typical of this stigma.
The colicky manifestations make the patient irritable. All
bowel and intestinal troubles of sycotic origin have the
constant symptom of colic, whether it be in the diarrhœa,
the hæmorrhoids, or any other digestive manifestation ;
and with this there is always the marked irritability.

The sycotic child is sour-smelling in all ways ; even the
stools smell sour. He wants constant attention ; he must be
rocked or carried ; his colics are > from lying on the abdomen
or from pressure. *Dulcamara* is typically sycotic in its
manifestations ; it has the diarrhœa, acrid and corrosive ;
from getting wet ; bleeding hæmorrhoids with great pruritis ;
fishbrine smell.

In the urinary tract there are many symptoms. There is
intense pain on urination ; children scream from the pain.
This is due to a spasmodic contraction affecting the urethra.
Many diseases of the urinary tract are combined syphilis,
psora and sycosis, with the last two most prominent. The
diabetic patient is usually strongly tubercular, but if there is
a sycotic taint as well, the condition becomes much more
malignant. Bright's disease is a manifestation of all three
stigmata combined. Where we find fibrous changes we may
be sure there is a strong sycotic influence.

In the rectum we find many conditions of tubercular
origin, as strictures, fistulæ, sinuses and pockets, but when
there is the addition of the sycotic stigma the conditions are
greatly aggravated, and there is much more tendency
toward malignancy, for combinations of the tubercular
diathesis with sycosis produce cancerous affections.

In acquired sycotic conditions represented by prostatic gland troubles there is a combination of all three stigmata. The most frequent location of the sycotic manifestations in women is in the pelvic organs. Pelvic inflammations such as inflammation of the ovaries, inflammatory processes of the fallopian tubes ; in fact, all of the inflammatory diseases of the female pelvis may be traced to this taint. In the more chronic types we get cystic degeneration of the ovaries, the uterus and the fallopian tubes. Again, the infection may pass on into the peritoneal cavity, and we find general peritonitis and general cellulitis. Appendicitis is directly traceable to sycotic influences.

To distinguish the sycotic manifestations in the abdomen, bear in mind the colicky, spasmodic and often paroxysmal pains of sycosis, the acrid discharges which corrode the skin ; the stale fish or fishbrine odour of the discharges ; the mottled appearance of the mucous membrane.

The attempt to suppress sycotic manifestations, especially the discharges, is very common medical practice ; but suppressive measures meet with a very prompt and decided renewal of the stigmatic power and energy. After such an attempt, the destructive progress of the disease becomes much more rapid, and often leads rapidly to malignancies. This is very often seen in the disturbances of the sexual organs which lead to surgery as a way out of the difficulty, and immediately after operation, when the physician has reason to believe his patient to be on the road to recovery, there will be a sudden flaring up of the difficulty and death ensues very soon. When such a series of circumstances occurs, it is unquestionably because of the sycotic influence that may have been more or less unnoticed in the patient's condition. Often there is such a sequence of events after some injury.

Sycosis, continuing the gonorrhœal poison in its chronic state, has the rheumatic conditions that we may expect. There are tearing pains in the joints, which are < during rest, < during cold damp weather, > moving or stretching, > dry weather. There are pains in the small joints with infiltrations and deposits. Stiffness, soreness and lameness are characteristic of this stigma. The troubles in the joints, where there are deposits of lime salts as in arthritis deformans, are sycotic. The gouty diathesis has a sycotic base.

The sycotic skin manifestations tend toward overgrowth or extra deposits. The nails are ribbed or ridged and thick and heavy. Moles, warts, wine-coloured patches and other manifestations of unnaturally thickened skin belong in this classification. Skin eruptions of this stigma occur in circumscribed spots, and there are exfoliating eczemas. Psoriasis is a combination of the three stigmata, with sycosis and psora predominating. The fishscale eruptions are also a combination of the three stigmata, with the dryness of psora, the squamous character of syphilis and the overgrowth of tissue, or the thickened skin manifestations, of sycosis. Herpes zoster has a sycotic base. Malignancies of the skin are more violent and intractable in proportion as the sycotic taint is increased. Barber's itch readily develops in sycotic patients, while it rarely develops unless there is a sycotic taint.

We have all noted the tendency of some operated patients to develop stitch abscesses. This never occurs unless there is a sycotic tendency in the patient.

Chapter XXX

SYCOSIS—OVER-CONSTRUCTION

When we come to analyse the sycotic miasm in relation to the table of elements and their respective atomic weights, we find an entirely new grouping of symptoms. We have stated in the summary of the miasmatic symptomatology that the psoric manifests most strongly the functional symptoms ; the syphilitic has as its hallmark ulceration and destruction of tissue, even to bony tissue ; while the sycotic has an opposite manifestation—infiltration and overgrowth of tissue.

Therefore we see that the sycotic stigma presents a problem in physical construction that is the exact opposite of the psoric, granting that our theory has been so far sound. Thus, while the psoric patient is unable to assimilate sufficient elements from sunlight, air, water, food, etc., for a well rounded physical structure in which to house a normal healthy mind and spirit, we find that the sycotic patient is too susceptible to the available constructive elements ; he seizes upon and assimilates to the point of overgrowth of tissues. If this is so, it explains the reason for pathology in all parts of the body that manifest overgrowth of natural tissue ; and we have already noted that where we find malignancies with overgrowth of tissues and infiltrations we are almost always able to trace the sycotic taint.

Consider the necessary elements for physical construction and the lavish manner in which they are supplied by Nature in fresh air, sunshine, fresh fruits, vegetables, nuts, even in fresh sea food and animal tissue which we adapt for food. In the case of manganese, for instance, McCollum tells us that but a small amount is required in our daily food, but that it is very difficult to prepare a diet entirely free from the element for experimental purposes. If it is so difficult to prepare food and omit the small amount required, what an excess of the substance must be available in a normal diet. Yet the healthy normal system absorbs only the amount required to maintain a state of health.

A list of antisycotic remedies has been compiled from several standard works on materia medica ; we shall give a list excerpted from this, comprising only those remedies with a primary chemical relationship. It will be noted that almost all these remedies fall within the group of body-construction elements ; but it is significant that the so-called "double salts" predominate. Another interesting fact is that the carbons are almost entirely lacking, while the Calcareas appear infrequently. Chemical combinations of the very lowest elements are found to be fairly frequent, as in *Fluoric acid, Nitric acid, Ammonium mur.* It is interesting to note that while there is a preponderance of the *Kali's*, *Kali carb.* is omitted. It will be noted, too, that while *Aurum mur., Baryta mur., Cinnabaris, Mercury* and *Plumbum* appear in this list, the first three are tinctured with elements of a much lower atomic weight, while the two last are comparatively rarely indicated in true sycotic conditions unless there is a syphilitic taint as well ; although of course these might be indicated when the condition approaches disintegration of tissue as toward the final chapter of the disease. Let us examine these remedies, comparing their relationships by number to the elements.

Alumina 13.	*Fluoric acid* 1, 9.
Ammonium mur. 1, 7, 17.	*Graphites* 6, 14, 26.
Antimony 51.	*Hepar sulph.* 16, 20.
Argentum 47.	*Kali bich.* 19, 24.
Arsenic 33.	*Kali iod.* 19, 53.
Aurum mur. 17, 79.	*Kali mur.* 17, 19.
Baryta mur. 17, 56.	*Kali sulph.* 16, 19.
Borax 1, 5, 8, 11.	*Lithium* 3.
Bismuth 33.	*Mercury* 80.
Bromium 35.	*Merc. cor.* 17, 80.
Calcarea phos. 15, 20.	*Merc. i. r.* 53, 80.
Cinnabaris 16, 80.	*Merc. sol.* 1, 7, 8, 80.
Chlorine 17.	*Natrum mur.* 11, 17.
Ferrum iod. 26, 53.	*Natrum sulph.* 11, 16.
Ferrum phos. 15, 26.	*Nitric acid* 1, 7, 8.

Phosphorus 15.   *Silica* 14.
Plumbum 82.   *Sulphur* 16.

It is not to be thought that these remedies, even with those from animal and vegetable sources added, are all that might be indicated in sycotic conditions ; but these show the trend of the remedies that are most likely to be indicated. It is an accepted fact that all plant remedies contain the constructive elements, rebuilt into potential and varied combinations in every species of plant life. So too our animal remedies have their value only in what has been made of the elements assimilated and rebuilt. It is this reconstruction that gives their potentiality.

However, in the association of elements with the remedies under consideration, we note a greater proportion of those containing chlorine (17) than any other element. Further, we note a gap between Bromine (53) and Argentum (47). In order of atomic weights the following fill in this space : Krypton 36 ; Rubidium 37 ; Strontium 38 ; Yttrium 39 ; Zirconium 40 ; Columbium 41 ; Molybdenum 42 ; undetermined 43 ; Ruthenium 44 ; Rhodium 45 ; Palladium 46. Of these Strontium and Palladium have had considerable provings, and both have been found useful in sycotic conditions. However, Strontium is found in natural association with Plumbum, and its greatest influence, homœopathically, seems to lie along similar lines. Palladium and Rhodium (the latter has had a brief proving) are associated in their natural state with Platinum ; the latter being in the higher register of atomic weights, we consider as being more particularly in the destructive classification. However, Cadmium (48) is a remedy to be considered in this antisycotic group, particularly in pathological end products.

Some of the elements that come within the range of the constructive group, yet which have never been defined as having constructive roles, have been detected by the spectrograph in milk ; these are : Barium 56 ; Boron 5 ; Lithium 3 ; Rubidium 37 ; Strontium 38 ; Titanium 22 ; Zinc 30 ; also, by other investigators, Aluminium 13 ; Chromium 24 ; Lead 82 ; Silicon 14 ; Tin 50 ; Vanadium 23 ; Manganese 25. These are by no means all the inorganic substances contained in milk, but are those that have been detected only in traces, and their constructive duties have not been defined.

Detection of these elements is of particular interest in that it suggests roles of some sort to elements heretofore missing in our constructive elements ; and because of its inclusion of Barium and Lead, the latter being so far beyond the constructive limits as we have understood them. Moreover, these elements, associated with physical functions of the body (albeit in animals) leads us to inquire why elements of such high atomic weight should appear in nutritional functions ? Was this by chance, some imperfection in technique on the part of the investigators, or have we a still wider field beyond that compassed by our present knowledge and the hypothesis founded thereon ?

These comments upon the remedies frequently associated by symptomatology with the problems of hereditary or contracted disease taints must be understood to be no more than the first uncertain steps toward a newer understanding of the relationship of our potentized remedies to cases that may present themselves before us. We realize it is far less important to rationalize the REASONS FOR than to embrace a knowledge of the means to CARE FOR these conditions ; but while these suggestions of the possible *modus operandi* of a certain group of elements are extremely rudimentary, it is hoped that the problems involved will be clarified by more study to the point where here, too, we may verify the whole process of logical reasoning and scientific procedure that has made homœopathy THE profoundly coherent system of healing.

CHAPTER XXXI

DISEASE CLASSIFICATION : A SUMMARY

LET us summarize the different stigmata, remembering that we may get all shadings of all the stigmata in their groupings in our patients, but one stigma will predominate above all the others. They all have their characteristic differences. The accentuation of psora is functional ; the accentuation of the syphilitic taint is ulcerative ; the accentuation of sycosis is infiltration and deposits.

When suppressed, the syphilitic stigma spends itself on the meninges of the brain, and affects the larynx and throat in general, the eyes, the bones and the periosteum.

Psora spends its action very largely upon the nervous system and the nerve centres, producing functional disturbances, which are > by surface manifestations.

Sycosis attacks the internal organs, especially the pelvic and sexual organs. In this stigma we find the worst forms of inflammation, infiltration of the tissues causing abscesses, hypertrophies, cystic degeneration ; when thrown back into the system by suppression this stigma causes dishonesty, moral degeneracy and mania.

In treating patients suffering from these stigmata. this classification is of inestimable value, for it immediately throws the *simillimum* into a class of remedies corresponding with the accentuation of the stigma that is outstanding in the case, and this should be considered in the totality ; it will often throw light upon the choice of a *simillimum* that is applicable to the individual case and stage of development.

When we are considering a case manifesting mixed stigmata, there is always one more prominent, and this will be the one requiring relief ; when this is relieved, the next in prominence must be cared for, until the patient is freed from the inheritance of generations.

Chapter XXXII

HOMŒOPATHIC THERAPEUTICS IN THE FIELD OF ENDOCRINOLOGY

THE viewpoint of the modern physiologist reflects the theory that the vast majority of human ills are traceable to dysfunctions of the glandular system ; that most growth problems (over- and under-development of the whole body or parts) and many maladjustments of the child to its environment, and even of the adult to his relationships and problems, are related in some degree to endocrine imbalance. The modern student of homœopathy may have learned to scoff at the philosophy of Hahnemann, yet how close the endocrinologist's findings are to the teachings of Hahnemann —that the human being is a unit, mind, body and spirit— and that these are so correlated as to act freely and without impediment when the vital principle, the spirit-like force or dynamis, is in equilibrium ; yet if this equilibrium of health be thrown out of balance by the dysfunction of one member (or if this imbalance be manifest by the dysfunction principally of one organ) the whole is affected to a greater or less degree.

So it is, also, that the function of some of the ductless glands is to secrete a minute quantity of specialized product into the system, a secretion that has a vital bearing on the health of the whole constitution. In many cases this secretion of a normal gland is so minute that it approaches the homœopathic attenuation.

With this concept of the importance of the endocrine glands in maintaining health, and with the almost infinitesimal amount of some of these glandular secretions, we can hardly fail to see the important relationship the homœopathic remedy may hold to the manifestations of endocrine dysfunction and to the balance of the ductless glands themselves.

In considering this vast subject it is apropos to quote

from the book by August A. Werner, M.D., F.A.C.P., entitled *Endocrinology* (Lea & Febiger, 1937) :

There has been much complaint from physicians in general that the literature on endocrinology is technical and difficult to understand. There are several reasons for these seeming difficulties, among which may be mentioned (1) the newness of the subject ; (2) the lack of definite information as to the possible number of hormones and their functions ; (3) the intricate inter- relationship of the secretions of the ductless glands ; (4) the difficulty in application of the results of animal experimentation to the human, which, aside from the scientific value of such work, is the ultimate object of these investigations ; (5) the variation of potency of the hormonal preparations used, and (6) the difficulty of determining individual dosage, which is influenced by the degree of function of the glands of the patient, the individual susceptibilities of the patient, cellular receptivity, interaction of other endocrine secretions, and the effect of general metabolic factors and disease processes in each individual. . . .

To be a good clinical endocrinologist, one must first be a good internist, and the time is not far distant when, in order to be a good internist, one must be a good endocrinologist. . . .

It is necessary to have :

1. A thorough knowledge of the anatomical structure and arrangement of the autonomic nervous system. Its division into two parts, viz. the parasympathetic and the sympathetic ; a knowledge of the function of these two divisions which are diametrically opposed to each other when stimulated.

2. Comprehension of the function of the endocrine glands, in so far as this has been definitely or reasonably established.

3. The recognition that the intricate vital life processes of the body over which we have no control, such as the regulation of normal growth and development, the digestion, absorption, and assimilation of food and its release from the storehouses, such as the liver and muscles for the production of energy, the continua- tion of cardiac action and respiration at a normal rate, our sense of well being ; all these and more, depend in great measure upon the maintenance of a delicate equilibrium between the two divisions of the autonomic nervous system.

4. A knowledge that the maintenance of this functional balance between the parasympathetic and sympathetic divisions of the autonomic nervous system is markedly influenced by the internal secretions of the ductless glands which act as governors over it. . . .

There is a great clamour from the medical profession for information on treatment of endocrine conditions. Before we can treat any abnormal condition successfully we must first have knowledge of the syndrome and its etiology (*here speaks the viewpoint of the orthodox school*) and secondly, we must have potent preparations for treatment. Many endocrine syndromes have been recognized in the past before active principles were available for treatment. This condition still exists and the possession of active hormones does not always insure that relief can be given, for obvious reasons. With the desire and urge to alleviate these endocrine syndromes, all manner of glandular preparations have been utilized, many of which are inert, especially when administered orally. . . ."

In closing his Preface Dr. Werner gives credit to various members of the profession who have been of great help to him, and speaks of one member with the following significant tribute :

Where an understanding of the fundamentals of endocrinology was acquired, and the lesson was inculca. .d to study the patient's condition with every conceivable relationship to disease in mind and not as an aggregation of glands.

In his first chapter the author cites the influence of emotions, as well as the reaction of various drugs, on various functions, with the reflex action on the glands through the nervous system. His comments on the organs in sickness and health recall Hahnemann's observations, but in this 1937 observation Dr. Werner does not achieve the practical application of Hahnemann's logic and philosophy which seems so plain to us.

However, even a brief survey of his work astonishes us with the wide range of syndromes which Dr. Werner suggests are caused by glandular dysfunctions or are influenced by glandular preparations. These conditions range from acne to hæmophilia, from anæmia to deformed and distorted skeletal formation in children or developing in adult life. This implies that a vast array, if not the majority, of constitutional afflictions are due to glandular dysfunction, and therefore we may assume that the constitutional homœopathic remedy will have its usefulness here in the light of modern knowledge just as it has had in the past when we did not realize the importance of a knowledge of endocrinology, but trusted to the totality of symptoms as our sure guide in prescribing.

There is little doubt that the majority of cases of over- and under-development of tissues or organs such as adiposis, obesity, inhibition of or precocious development of sex characteristics (whether traceable to the pineal, pituitary or thyroid glands or the gonads), and changes in the skeleton formation such as may come from dysfunction of the parathyroid, are, in the language of Hahnemann, manifestations of the miasms, either inherited or acquired. It may be circumstantial evidence for the miasm theory that certain types of manifestations are found among certain peoples, just as the types of obesity which are found largely in the Hebrew race ; for one might argue with equal weight that centuries of prescribed diet might have had its influence. Nevertheless, in many cases of glandular dysfunction we are able to trace like tendencies through a family history. Sometimes in a case where no such evidence is available we may find a history, or definite evidence, of venereal infection, very often reported as cured by scientific treatment.

To the Hahnemannian homœopath, the lack of laboratory corroboration has little weight because he realizes that the miasm may persist after the organism has been suppressed, diminished or destroyed by treatments in the infected individual or by passing through successive generations.

In any case, while the orthodox school works on the basis of the objective symptoms, merely recognizing as concomitants the subjective symptoms which to them are extraneous for clinical purposes (even while they acknowledge their theoretically correct glandular extracts as inert !) the homœopathic school fixes its attention on the individual's subjective manifestations in accordance with Hahnemann's logical development of the therapeutic principle.

Such a book as Dr. Werner's offers us the most up-to-date discussions on the pathology, etiology and diagnosis of these conditions, but there is little real help here in the therapeutic field. Let us turn to such a book for such information as we may glean from the modern authors and research workers, but let us turn to a study of our rich fund of materia medica and philosophy when we wish to help the patient toward cure.

As an index to our cumbersome materia medica let us turn to our repertories with the constitutional symptoms of the sick individual in mind. Here we are not forced to trace the organ supposedly responsible for the manifestations in the patient ; instead, we note the symptoms peculiar to the patient—symptoms mental and physical—and by meeting the symptoms of the individual with the corresponding symptoms of the indicated remedy we shall be able to meet like with like, and with reasonable assurance we can test the homœopathic principle in these as in other cases.

Of course it is necessary in these cases, as in all others, to consider the possibility of cure, just as Hahnemann taught. This is well summed up in the concluding paragraph of an editorial in the October 1938 issue of the *British Homœopathic Journal*, which we quote :

In estimating the possibility of successful homœopathic treatment of deficiency diseases we must, of course, recognize that the action of drugs is by eliciting a response from a living cell ; they cannot do this from those that are dead or restore them to life. It is of no use to attempt the impossible. But we should also recognize that no organ or tissue becomes suddenly destroyed, unless it be by trauma, and that there are all degrees of failure of function, and if the failure has not gone too far it should be, and we believe it is, possible to restore it to the normal by the giving of the simillimum. . . . To this end we need a deeper acquaintance with our remedies. We are using practically the same materia medica that we did fifty or more years ago. It requires no alteration, but it does need to be added to, not by the addition of more remedies, . . . but by fresh provings to pursue the action of our drugs into the realm of modern physiological research, and especially their action on the endocrine organs. If we do not increase our knowledge of the capabilities of our drugs our homœopathic art will become static. It will make no progress.

It was our purpose to suggest several rubrics from both the Kent and Bœnninghausen repertories that are peculiarly pertinent to the conditions we are studying, but when we were brought face to face with the widely varying array of functional symptoms manifested by these patients, it seems we can do no more than commend to you the repertories themselves, and advise the physician who wishes to cure his patient not to neglect these valuable adjuncts to successful prescribing. In other words, when a cursory glance at a modern work on endocrine dysfunction covers such a wide range of symptoms, it is impossible to limit the possible symptoms in even a few syndromes. Again and again we are faced with the conviction that we are dealing with what we have already long since learned to know as constitutional symptoms, and we cannot think of a few rubrics that might be useful without omitting others even more valuable. So we can only repeat : Learn the value of your repertory for reference work, and you will be well repaid for the time expended.

Nor can we, in one brief paper, begin to consider the syndromes which we meet in daily practice, and which we recognize as having endocrine relationships. We may only sketch a few of these conditions with a very restricted consideration of suitable therapeutic measures ; and we may briefly outline a few outstanding remedies having general influence on glandular structure.

Probably the type of glandular imbalance we meet most frequently is diabetes mellitus. The accepted therapy is insulin, and it has a definite influence on the sugar output ; yet few physicians pause to consider whether this treatment is curative or merely palliative—a substitution therapy. Recent experiments indicate that continued massive doses of insulin may result in an increase of sugar following an initial decrease ; and that it may remain at a fairly high level so long as the insulin therapy is pushed. A case recently observed provided the interesting phenomenon of a marked decrease of sugar output when the patient was forced to do without her insulin for a few days ; and that when she returned to a decreased insulin dosage the amount of sugar remained at a much lower level than while she was receiving massive doses. A series of observations on patients under homœopathic care would be valuable.

We must remember that once insulin therapy is established, it tends to become necessary to the patient and there is little hope of establishing normal balance. Therefore it is more practical to begin treatment by the use of the homœopathic remedy, for we can always go to insulin later if this is necessary. We find suitable remedies for *Sugar in Urine* in the repertories, and most of the remedies listed are deep in action or are closely related to emotional states. The diabetic patient usually presents subjective symptoms that clearly indicate the *simillimum*, or he may be able to give a history of emotional shock preceding his present affliction that will point the way to the remedy. It is possible that his symptoms are so clearly marked that the indications for a constitutional remedy cannot be overlooked, even though his remedy has not been proven to produce the sugar imbalance. In such case, if the patient improves on the indicated remedy, we are justified in adding it to those already listed, giving it a tentative clinical rating. If the general level of health is raised, even though the low sugar threshold remains the same, we may safely rely on the remedy which maintains general improvement, and not be too anxious over the sugar output.

Recent research work has indicated the influence of the pancreas in peptic ulcer. There is probably no surgical condition which yields so readily to the homœopathic remedy and proper diet, if it is discovered before surgery is necessary to save life. These conditions usually present enough subjective symptoms to define the *simillimum* from the list of suitable remedies Kent gives ; in this list, too, we find the polychrests to the fore, probably with the *Kali's*, *Lycopodium* and *Phosphorus* leading.

It is frequently the case that in exploratory operations the close prescriber finds evidence of ulcers healed under his earlier prescriptions—in other words, homœopathic prescribing has left its signature on diseased tissues.

Another frequent exhibition of endocrine imbalance is the disturbances of the menopause. These patients give us a wealth of subjective symptoms. In fact, many of these women are so voluble that we cannot overlook that great leader among the many indicated remedies for this particular state in life—*Lachesis*. But a well-rounded symptom analysis may show us some other remedy to have greater applicability.

Hyperæmesis gravidarum is a serious condition we meet occasionally. If this condition is met early enough and we can find the indicated remedy, neither surgery nor yet endocrine preparations will be required. In the July 1938 *Homœopathic Recorder* Dr. Allan D. Sutherland gives us the indications for *Ars.*, *Bry.*, *Cocc.*, *Colch.*, *Kali c.* (the sudden nausea coming on while walking and the sudden overpowering sleepiness after eating a mouthful or two) ; *Nat. mur.*, *Petr.*, *Phos.*, *Sulph.*, *Verat. a.* Many of us do not think so often of *Aletris farinosa* with its muscular atony and chlorotic history. We would add to Dr. Sutherland's list the nosodes, *Medorrhinum*, *Psorinum*, *Syphillinum* and *Tuberculinum*, for consideration. Dr. Sutherland is careful to point out that this is but a brief list of the possibilities ; but it is valuable as a suggestion of help in critical conditions.

One of the most distressing conditions we have to deal with (and one we fortunately rarely meet) is enlarged thymus. In his discussion of this condition, Werner states his conviction that it is not the enlargement of the gland itself which causes the sudden death, but that this condition is concomitant to the influence of the vagus nerve on the heart. This indicates even more strongly the necessity for the constitutional remedy for the small child, and the physician must be keen in watching his development, for all too often the child is in apparently good health until attacked suddenly and without warning. Where cyanosis, suffocative attacks or other symptoms occur, however slight, a remedy may be found that will carry the child through to normal health. If the symptoms take an asthmatic tendency we have more assurance in selecting the constitutional remedy.

In general practice we frequently meet children who are backward in mind and body. Here is a field where we are able to do remarkably good work with our remedies. The *Barium* salts are not sufficiently appreciated for such work, but the *Calcarea* group, *Silica* or *Sulphur* (to mention but a few) may be more clearly indicated. Even the *Kalis* and the *Natrums* are surprisingly successful when indicated. When the constitutional remedy is found, it is surprising how these children—under-developed, dull, stupid, unable to learn, perhaps nervous and high-strung—react to normal development.

Often these children are deceitful as well as·backward ; then we add *Arg. nit.* and perhaps *Bufo* to our list ; and if they are convulsive children these remedies may be even more strongly indicated.

A consideration of the mental and emotional states is our best indication for the *simillimum*. This is not as simple as to feed glandular preparations, perhaps, but it is less apt to throw other glandular secretions out of proportion, and the results seem to be generally better. And no man who has watched the action of our potencies can doubt their efficacy.

To a large extent the remedies which come to mind as constitutional remedies of sufficient depth to influence these glandular conditions with their structural and nervous concomitants are our great polychrests, and many of these are from the same chemical base as the elements of the physical body—*Sulphur, Silica, Phosphorus, Kali, Natrum,* the *Carbons.* Then we find such remedies as *Lycopodium, Nitric acid,* and the major nosodes, of great use in these conditions. It is impossible, as well as dangerous practice, to name leading remedies for any pathological condition, and still more for any functional disturbance ; yet there are valuable remedies which have a wide range and frequent usage in our daily practice that are not so valuable in these conditions.

In running over suitable rubrics for glandular conditions we find *Pulsatilla* conspicuous by its absence in many rubrics, and when it occurs it is in the lower ratings. On the other hand, we find *Lycopodium* is a leader. *Lycopodium* is one of the very few survivors from the first era of plant life, and it has changed very little in appearance. It has survived because of the basic qualities inherent in the development of all life, and probably, therefore, has a greater potential influence on organic functions.

There is hardly an organ or function that is not influenced by that greatest of all polychrests, *Sulphur.* Even Hering noted its influence on such glandular conditions as were then recognized. We have spoken of its value in developing backward children. It is classical for its use in deep-seated affections resulting from the suppression of superficial symptoms. It has proven its usefulness in diabetes mellitus. We all know the classical indications for *Sulphur* ; but in passing it briefly, we mention one function of *Sulphur* we may have occasion to invoke : that of stirring the organism to reaction when other seemingly indicated remedies fail to act, especially if there are recurrences of acute or subacute manifestations—where the patient moves toward recovery only to slip back repeatedly.

Phosphorus resembles *Sulphur* in its fields of usefulness as in many of its symptoms, while being quite different in its classical constitution. Where *Sulphur* is indolent, *Phosphorus* is over-excitable, erotic in many manifestations and erratic in most symptoms related to the sexual functions. These manifestations range from insanity or lascivious ideas to vicarious menstruation, impotence and abnormal labours. *Phosphorus* affects the development of the physical body in the child, his ability to concentrate his mental efforts, and the normal functioning of the adult, just as in *Sulphur*. Prostrated energies from loss of fluids and from emotional and physical strain are characteristic of *Phosphorus*, as against the general lack of energy in *Sulphur*.

Both *Phosphorus* and *Phosphoric acid* are to be considered in glycosuria, as well as other glandular difficulties.

Nitric acid has a powerful action on glandular dysfunctions, especially of syphilitic origin, although it is antipsoric and antisycotic as well. Sensitiveness is a keynote of this remedy—of the head or of affected parts, to touch, jars, sudden motion or sudden change in tempo of motion; to cold, to changes in the weather; tendency to take cold. There is great disturbance of the circulation ; the fingers and toes appear livid, pale, cold or dead at times. The characteristic sensation as of a splinter in the affected parts, particularly in such tissues as the tonsils, is found also in *Arg. nit.* and *Hepar*. In *Nitric acid* the disturbance of the sexual organs and functions rivals *Phosphorus*, and sometimes there is almost as much lasciviousness. In general the sensitiveness and excitability is uppermost, but they tire quickly ; old people calling for this remedy manifest excessive prostration.

" Vegetable *Sulphur* ", or *Lycopodium*, is one of the great trio of remedies (*Sulphur*, *Calcarea* and *Lycopodium*) about which, as Clarke says, " all the rest of the materia medica can be grouped ". Like the rest of the trio, it has swollen glands, and is one of the few specifically mentioned as having goitre. Acute glandular affections start on the right side and tend to move to the left. This is one of the few remedies mentioned in the materia medica as definitely tending to enlargement of bony tissue, whereas *Phosphorus* tends to thickening of bony tissue. Characteristically, *Lycopodium* has a furrowed face and forehead ; thin face and neck and perhaps upper chest, while he remains plump below, or there is progressive emaciation from above downward. Great weariness and lassitude, especially in the legs after slight exertion, and great want of bodily heat ; deadness of the fingers and hands as in *Nitric acid* ; he feels as if circulation were suspended. Mentally he is as fearful as *Phosphorus* and the *Kalis*, as sad as *Nitric acid* and the *Natrums* ; the burning pains make us think of the burnings of *Sulphur* and *Phosphorus*. Probably *Lycopodium* is the most flatulent remedy we shall consider, unless it be *Carbo veg.*, which has more heartburn.

The general state of gloominess and mental depression characterizes the *Natrum* group and is their great earmark in chronic states ; they almost delight to make themselves and others miserable by looking on the dark side ; strong aversion to consolation ; sometimes alternate gaiety and gloom.

These salts are a startling exposition of the power of potentization, for in this form they have the most profound action on the mental state, on physical functions, on the chemistry of fluids and the pathology of the organs. There is sudden failing of strength, excessive draining of body fluids coming on suddenly, sudden depletion of the sexual organs because of excessive stimulation ; rapid changes in the blood ; sudden and profound emaciation, often following previous increase of flesh. *Nat. mur.* particularly, emaciates about the neck, even when eating ravenously. This group of remedies affects the thyroid gland markedly, and has the subjective sensation of compression, as if there were a lump or plug in the throat. *Nat. ars.* has the sensation as if the thyroid body were compressed between the thumb and finger. *Nat. carb.* has the hard swelling of the thyroid.

Clarke tells us, in his *Dictionary*, that *Nat. carb.* gives the type of the family group, while *Nat. mur.* is the most important remedy of the group, ranking with the polychrests.

These remedies are exceedingly sensitive to cold ; *Nat. carb.* is the chilliest ; it cannotst and cold air, draughts, cannot stand a change of clothing or a drink of cold water because of the chill ; yet *Nat. carb.* is unable to stand the heat of the sun and succumbs easily to heat stroke. He has no physical stamina ; he exhausts quickly from mental or bodily exertion, and suffers great debility. Like the family, he is profoundly exhausted after a short walk, and *Nat. carb.* particularly suffers from the effects of overstudy. The nervous system is weak yet is easily affected almost to hysteria, just as in the sexual sphere there is sterility because of over-activity of the organs.

Other outstanding manifestations of the exceedingly sensitive state of the nervous system is the extreme sensitivity to music and the aggravation therefrom, and the aggravation before and during electrical storms. Like all the *Natrums*, there is anæmia with an increase in the white cells and decrease of red cells ; with this there is emaciation and bloating. Children find walking difficult because of even weaker ankles than in *Sulphur* ; they are disinclined to study because it is so exhausting ; nervous almost to hysteria ; pale, weak, easily tired, easily chilled ; they bore their fingers into ears and nose and it seems to relieve. The adult *Nat. carb.* patient shows much the same picture, but if a man, he tends toward priapism ; if a woman, there is a discharge of mucus and the semen after coition with consequent sterility ; if she goes on to gestation, labour pains are weak and ineffectual and she begs for massage. The *Nat. carb.* patient is always spraining a wrist, an ankle, a knee, dislocating a joint or straining a muscle in the back.

Nat. hypochlorosum is distinguished from the others of the family group by its rapid emaciation with a sudden, waterlogged uterus which sags into the lower pelvis with the sensation as if it would fall out ; with this there is almost a globus hystericus which seems to rise from the uterus into the upper chest. Faintness, weakness and weariness, so that she falls asleep whenever she sits down, with flabbiness and a diffused hydrogenoid condition with a tendency to leucocytosis mark this remedy.

It is difficult to confine oneself to a brief outline of *Nat. mur.* Clarke tells us that it corresponds to that type of constipation which is associated with anæmia, chilliness (especially down the back) and cold feet ; or to indigestion in masturbators. The degree of melancholy keeps pace with the constipation, just as in *Nat. sulph.* the melancholy keeps step with the degree of indigestion.

Tears are a keynote of *Nat. mur.* : tears with the emotional depression, tears even with the laughter, for she laughs until she weeps at things not at all funny ; tears with the coryza, and even with the whooping-cough. The face is earthy, dirty and greasy. The strong desire for salt is even more marked in the nausea and vomiting of pregnancy. In adults suffering from glandular imbalance, with a history of malarial fever and the classic dosing of quinine, *Nat. mur.* may unlock the case and even carry it to cure. The *Nat. mur.* child is slow in learning to walk and talk, craves salt so that he will eat it as some children do sweets, and when out of doors is apt to eat earth. We are told that *Nat. mur.* is the chronic of *Ignatia* ; certainly the emotional *Natrum* family shows the effects of emotional strain or shock as much as *Ignatia* ; and *Ignatia*, by the way, is a remedy we often overlook in diabetes following emotional shock.

Nat. phos. children develop improperly because of excess of lactic acid in their diet. It merits wider use than it has received, and its general features are marked by the parent substances. Like *Phosphorus*, it is effective in diabetes, but here it shows its relationship to the *Natrums*, because this diabetes is apt to be a reflex of hepatic derangement. There is much disturbance of the sexual organs ; there is weak back and trembling limbs, especially knees, after coition and after the nightly involuntary emissions. Instead of the weak, lax muscles of *Nat. carb.* we find here a tension of muscles. There is inability to apply himself to his books, and even the effort causes despondency.

Nat. sulph. is unusually gloomy, even for this gloomy family. It is strongly hydrogenoid in tendency ; there is marked aggravation from water and dampness ; he may be so sensitive to this that he cannot eat food grown on wet ground ; he cannot live with comfort near a body of water. *Nat. sulph.* has less influence on goitre, perhaps, but there is the sense of constriction in the throat that foreshadows its usefulness in this field. It has marked usefulness in the enlargement of the liver and spleen and is almost as useful in old malarias as *Nat. mur.* It is particularly valuable in glandular imbalance following injuries to the head ; in fact, it is almost a specific for head injuries, even long after the trauma. It has profound action on the blood, and it has proved its usefulness in leukæmia.

In his *Dictionary* Clarke lists twenty-one *Kalis*, the majority having been well proven. T. F. Allen said the *Kali* salts were insidious in action and destructive of every organ and tissue in the body, so it is natural they are frequently indicated in glandular dysfunction.

No doubt the predominant action of the group is anti-syphilitic. There are the manifestations of primary syphilis, ulceration of mucous membranes, even destruction of bony structure as in the nose, as well as other symptoms of the miasm. On the other hand there is the marked sycotic trend as shown by the catarrhal discharges, and it has a field in acute gonorrhœa.

The chronic *Kali* patient exhibits the classical stature of the sycotic—rather short than tall, chubby to obesity, and with an accompanying anæmia. Here we have the perfect field for homœopathic therapeutics in endocrine imbalance, for there is a wealth of characteristic mental symptoms varying from the dull mentality with loss of memory and inability to exert the mind, even to softening of the brain, through all the states of nervous excitability (with or without intelligent co-ordination) to the high-strung nervous patient who borders on insanity or is actually insane. These people are easily startled at the slightest noise ; fearful, apprehensive, expect to die shortly and fear death. They may be as sad as the *Natrums* at times, but they are even more fearful. The *Natrums* have aggravation from mental exertion, but the *Kalis* cannot concentrate enough to bring on an aggravation.

Clinically, the following brief summary suggests fields of special usefulness in glandular dysfunctions, and indicates further study :

Kali aceticum in diabetes. *Kali arsenicum* for exophthalmic goitre. They are quarrelsome, discontented, jealous; the mental symptoms recur every third day.

Kali bromatum and *Kali phos.* are the most mentally degenerate of the *Kalis* ; both have developed softening of the brain in their clinical picture. Both remedies have done good work in the backward children and the aged. In the adolescent *Kali brom.* is often useful for acne appearing at that period. *Kali brom.* is useful in diabetes ; emissions, impotence and masturbation ; and in women, affections of the ovaries. *Kali brom.'s* peculiar mental symptom is that, when walking, he is sure he cannot pass a certain point ahead of him.

Kali phos. has marked flushing, especially in young people—they flush and pale because of nervousness and it aggravates the nervous strain. There is marked anæmia ; disturbance of the menstrual function ; atrophy of the male organs ; nymphomania. Sexual excitement, either indulged or suppressed, aggravates all symptoms.

Kali carb. is such a polychrest that it is difficult to limit it to a brief citation without omitting salient points. However, it is marked by such a great weariness that she wants to lie down, even in the street. It is exceedingly useful in the menopause, in disorders of pregnancy and in disordered menstrual functions. It is anæmic and obese, with atony of the muscles.

Kali ferrocyanatum deserves a wider use than it has received. It was well proven by Bell, who found that " it rivals *Sepia* in the uterine sphere ". These people are chlorotic and debilitated ; they suffer from dysmenorrhœa, dyspepsia and fatty degeneration of the heart—an exemplification of Allen's estimate of the family.

Kali iod. is one of our great goitre remedies and it also has atrophy of testes and mammae. Life seems insupportable to this patient ; he awakens at night to dread the return of dawn.

Kali mur. is the outstanding member of this family for swollen glands ; in fact, swelling is one of its characteristics, for it is very useful in swellings following blows, cuts and bruises. It may be indicated in glandular troubles following vaccination, and in Hodgkin's disease. The *Kalis* tend to white mucous surfaces, and *Kali mur.* is perhaps the most marked for this symptom.

Silica has such a vital relationship to growth, development and functions of mind and body that it is difficult to limit our view of it to brief mention. It affects the development of the bony structure and teeth, and is useful in knitting tissues after operation or trauma, or in removing keloid or abnormal scar tissue. There is profound action on the blood, and this, together with its affinity for glandular swellings, is the key to its suppurative tendency. A weak spine, brain fag, feeble circulation, caries, abscesses and fistulas, hernias and even hydrocele, give some idea of its depth and breadth of action. This is one of the few remedies listed as clinically useful in elephantiasis. Remember that vaccination or suppressed footsweat may be the cause of your *Silica* condition, and that your *Silica* child is the classic problem " angel child ".

The *Calcarea* group should be studied in these conditions. *Calcarea carb.*, especially, has a strong resemblance in the childhood symptoms to *Silica*, but where *Silica* has the suppurative tendency in glandular symptoms, *Calcarea's* tendency is to indurate. *Calcarea* is apt to be pot-bellied ; but there is the same depraved appetite as in *Silica*, a like relationship to growth and development of the teeth and bony structure, and as much anæmia, and even more spinal affections. It has the weak ankles and the child walks late ; the child is fat, rickety, pale, and sweats profusely about the head. *Calcarea's* sexual organs are greatly disturbed functionally, while *Silica's* sexual organs are apt to be more disturbed by pathology. *Calcarea* is the corpulent adult with full, even pendulous, abdomen and goitre or renal calculi.

We should remember the carbons—*Carbo veg.*, *Carbo an.*, *Graph.*, *Sepia*—in glandular conditions. The major nosodes merit further study along these lines, also. In fact, all our polychrests and many of our near-polychrests will yield richly to our search for effective remedies in endocrine disorders.

As homœopathic physicians, we have undertaken a labour that is vast in its expanse, yet it yields to us in the degree to which we apply ourselves in its pursuit. Our resources are far greater than those of the orthodox school ; we have proved them to be potent in a varying range of attenuations to suit best each man's experience and requirements. Our remedies will not upset the balance of endocrine secretions, for the *simillimum* will fill the demands of the system in all its parts without stimulating too much those organs which have maintained a relatively secure balance. In other words, our remedies affect directly the vital energy which in itself establishes equilibrium, those parts which are susceptible because of imbalance becoming a part of the normal healthy functioning of the whole unit.

Let us watch with great interest the investigation of the endocrine system, but let us look with the expectant eye of the explorer upon our homœopathic remedies, that we may meet and cure even these little-understood conditions.

CHAPTER XXXIII

THE PHENOMENOLOGICAL VIEWPOINT

In his introduction to his book, *Philosophy and the Concepts of Modern Science* (1935), Oliver L. Reiser, Associate Professor of Philosophy, University of Pittsburgh, tells us that the one possible method of :

. . . integrating the vast and unwieldly masses of facts of the sciences into meaningful wholes the adoption of a phenomenological viewpoint is recommended. By phenomenology is meant a study of that which exhibits or displays itself : it is the descriptive point of view obtained by viewing the thing as a whole. Much of the trouble . . . comes from an overemphasis upon microscopic details. Thus it comes about that we can no longer see the forest for the trees.

One of the really great discoveries of recent times is what has been termed the principle of *uniformitarianism* by the geologists ; that is, the theory that the forces now at work are identical in nature with those that produced changes in past ages.

If we take this phenomenological view of science to-day, we cannot help but see that Reiser's comment on the overemphasis upon microscopic details as being the source of multiplied data and chaotic theories of cause, action and effect is all too true. The strain of application to the microscope has produced a mental and philosophical astigmatism that permits each part to attain disproportionate focus in the whole.

Medicine, in particular, needs to view the whole and to take into consideration the principle of uniformitarianism. So far, as has been acknowledged by eminent authorities in the dominant school, homœopathy alone has offered such a unified theory that embraces the cause of diseased conditions, the course of the condition and its prognosis ; and at the same time the method of approach to the remedial agent, and the prognosis of its action upon the patient based upon the knowledge of the patient, the knowledge of the remedy, and a comprehension of the laws and their expression in varying states of health and disease. This is another way of saying that the homœopathic concept of disease and cure is from the phenomenological viewpoint in that it considers the broad outlines of the whole rather than some of the minute divisions compassed by microscopic vision, and at the same time embraces the meaning of which the microscopic vision demonstrates but a part.

It is safe to say that the revelations in science yet to come are even more vital and far-reaching than those already exhibited. The specialist in specific branches of medical investigation can furnish us vast and detailed information based on his microscopic findings ; yet as homœopathic physicians we cannot permit ourselves to be hampered by details to the exclusion of the whole. We are privileged to view all these findings as a part of the universal application of a Law under which we work ; for Man is naught if he be not a part of the Universe and subject to its laws.

Because man's adaptation is highly specialized, we are able to correlate, through a study of his health variations and the fundamental laws of the universe (as far as we can determine these), our knowledge of each toward greater comprehension and applicability of the greater to the individual problem. Animal life, like vegetable life, has a high degree of adaptability to environment and proves the most delicate laboratory we have for our examination ; yet the mineral kingdom furnishes us with an unsuspected link in our chain of evidence. Thus in conformity with statistical laws, we find again and again that the regular reaction or response of an individual is true of a group of individuals (with the necessary deductions for personal idiosyncrasies) and further, that what is true of a group of individuals may be true of any other group *in nature under similar conditions*, so far as we can measure the reactibility of these other groups. This uniformity of results is unquestionably due to what we term Universal Energy, which may be expressed again in very modern terms as those basic electrons, protons, neutrons, which are radiate, electric, magnetic—the very definition of potential energy. While energy has a certain stability of reactivity, it has selective action. Every portion of the human frame has a selective action over its function : it is susceptible to certain influences, constructive and destructive, and reacts selectively. Each atom of the human frame has a potential susceptibility to certain influences, and has developed selectively and according to the principles of uniformitarianism ; and we are now by no means in a static condition, socially, economically or physically, any more than the geological formation of the present day is in a static condition, *although both man and rocks may seem to be.*

In reality, we are continually in balance between dynamical laws and statistical laws, which are defined by Reiser as follows :

This duality of natural law is stated in terms of contrast between *dynamical* and *statistical* laws. The first type, *dynamical* laws, are *causal* laws, giving rigid determination and predictability, and the second type, *statistical* laws, yield more probability and introduce indeterminism into the calculations. A dynamical or causal law eliminates contingency, and implies ability to visualize the mechanisms in operation. But in statistical laws, concerned with the calculation of mean values, the individual elements of the statistical ensemble are not studied. . . . The atomic processes of microscopic mechanisms are reversible (sometimes periodically) and subject to necessary causal laws, whereas the macroscopic states represent the mean value of a large number of individual processes of a statistical aggregate. . . .

It is in this balance between dynamical and statistical laws that we find our margin of error in the application of homœopathic principles to our patients. The Law of Least Action is one of the dynamical laws upon which homœopathy was postulated and by which it has been affirmed. We acknowledge this law along with the Law of Similars and various other causal elements having to do with basic and cyclic action in natural processes, which in turn explain the processes of homœopathic action.

It has been argued that if homœopathy is the application of natural laws, the results of our remedies should be uniform ;

there should be less variation in the details of provings ; the length of action of any potency should be the same in all cases. No matter how careful the practitioner may be, he knows from bitter experience his failures, in spite of the most careful study and prescribing. There is no satisfaction in asserting that it is the failure of the prescriber ; it is unsatisfactory to accept the statement that variation in living conditions may be the cause. We can allow a margin for hereditary tendencies, and again for psychic or other forces which we understand too little, that govern the threads of our life span ; but beyond all this there are factors in the variation of remedy action that we are unable to understand. We may say that statistical laws authorize us to expect certain results from those dynamical laws which we attempt to utilize ; that in turn these statistical laws presuppose conditions pre-existing and perhaps unknown to us. But we may say, with more truth, that our incomplete understanding of dynamical laws causes us to assume statistical laws because it is a comfortable and convenient excuse ; our danger here lies in practising empiricism because of our dependence upon statistical laws.

Certainly we know that we have a variable force with which to deal in treating the sick. On the other hand, we question whether we have not a variable force with which to deal in our remedies. If the impulse of a force is equal to the change of momentum produced by it, as we are told in physics, we prove the power of our potentized remedies after administration by the clinical evidence, in direct proportion to the production of symptoms on the healthy human being.

Perhaps it is unfortunate that we have no measurable record of sickness or health, *per se.* There is no determinable level of health. Our imperfect senses are incapable of perfect registration or infallible translation of symptoms. Our probability of error is doubled when we deal with another, the sick individual. We review our results by the chemical formula : *The velocity of reaction is equal to the driving force divided by the resistance*—unfortunately we cannot know with precision either the actual driving force or the resistance.

Yet within certain limited fields we begin to measure the reactibility of the substances—animal, vegetable, mineral—

that form the basis of our potencies. Elementary work of this nature has been carried on, but it is far from having been perfected. It is enough to recognize that within the atom lies the solution to the problem of reaction of the various potencies. This is like stating that the atom is in structure much like the structure of the universe, and that the composition of the atom, like the universe, is made up of a similar " solar system " with planetary revolutions in their orbits. We draw the analogy that the atom offers the solution to universal physics, and that the universe itself offers aid in understanding our specific problems. Surely this is a phenomenological view of the homœopathic field !

Nevertheless, we suggest that these peculiarly pertinent questions are not elementary physics or chemistry ; they partake of universal breadth and embrace our very reasons for existence.

Consider again the question of potency. This has been a stumbling-block to many since Hahnemann's development of potentization. Modern science teaches that energy is automatically thrown off in proportion to the weight of the atom ; those of high atomic weight—radioactive—give off their own peculiar energy in proportionately high degree, destroying themselves in the process. If the atomic weight is lower, there is less intrinsic radiation and it becomes necessary to apply force to release the energy, until, in the low atomic weights more energy may be required to release the potential energy than thrift warrants, the erg unit being the expended effort and result. Yet for curative purposes it is probable that we might find the raw atom (as we may express it) entirely unfitted for our uses, and that the energy expended to break up the atomic structure sufficiently to release the electric, electromagnetic and magnetic orbits into malleable form for our purpose to be a sound investment of time and effort.

Consider lime and its various material uses ; consider how ineffective for physiological construction it is in its crude form, and indeed, how often it promotes rickets in children when introduced as lime water into the feeding formula. On the other hand, for countless conditions besides rachitic patients the homœopathic physician could ill afford to be without potentized calcium ; and infinitesimal amounts exhibit astoundingly curative results.

Recent developments in the study of the vitamins have demonstrated that in the lower trituations these become well-nigh inert, but by raising them to higher potencies in fluid form their activity and potent influence is markedly increased.

This leads us to meditate upon the comparative value of trituration and succussion as a means of stimulating the atom to a release of energy. It is impossible, of course, to attack the atom of lime by the same measures one employs to attack the molecular formation of plants. In some substances it is imperative to break down the bulk by trituration, while others are soluble in liquid and thus approach the state where the potential energy may be most readily released. If we were able to view the actual composition of the atom and its permeability, we might gain a fair idea of the reasons for energy release under different methods. This problem is allied equally to the construction of the atom and its destruction, with the result of wresting from it the greatest possible degree of its peculiar and intrinsic energy.

In viewing our potencies, we find the statistical laws govern in materia medica when we casually assume that remedy provings in the lower dilutions will be applicable in equal degree and unvaryingly, in the highest potencies. Again, we assume that any potency, say the 200th, is always to be depended upon for uniform results, in spite of widely varying methods of development. To be sure, experience has taught us that certain remedies have certain symptoms, which are more or less fixed in all provings and which act with greater or less regularity—sufficient as a basis for statistical observations—when applied clinically. Herein lies our art in homœopathy, but just here we lay ourselves open to criticism as being the scientists we claim to be.

Millikan tells us that under bombardment by alpha rays, an element may be built up to a higher atomic level ; at the same time neutrons may be thrown off, as a by-product of artificial transmutation. " These neutrons are presumably constituents of all nuclei except hydrogen, and many nuclear transformations throw them out." Neutrons carry no electrical charge, yet they are themselves weapons that may be hurled into atomic targets, making the atom unstable. This instability tends to step the atom down one degree and a proton—nucleus of hydrogen—flies out. Millikan tells us further that the neutron does not require great energy to get into a nucleus to transform it ; if it does so with violence the result is to shatter the nucleus and thus produce several substances of smaller atomic weight than the struck nucleus itself. On the other hand, it tends to " fall in . . . more easily and oftener when they have slow speeds than when they try to force their way in with violence. . . . In this way it adds its mass to that of the nucleus, so that the process results in the quiet building up of a heavier atom."

So far no technique has been devised to determine what the relation of trituration and succussion to energy release really means to the homœopathic preparation of remedies ; whether we actually change the character of the elements with which we deal, and if so, whether or not this is in a fixed ratio, is a problem for the homœopathic physicist. This is a field not yet developed, but one that offers a challenge to homœopathy. Here is an open question to intrigue the mind of science, a problem that, if solved in its elementary aspects, would place homœopathic principles on a footing with the field attained by the foremost scientific pioneers in physics !

Here we are faced with another problem in physics which has to do with the single remedy or polypharmacy. There is a reason for the single remedy even more profound than that practical one first advanced by Hahnemann and his followers : that since we know from careful provings what the single remedy will do, we can depend upon its uniformity (within certain limitations), but no one can predict the action of more than one remedy in combination or in alternation or in close proximity to each other. This is an observation, not an explanation.

Modern physics may give us the solution in the " wandering neutron " ; and neutrons are evidently loosed when certain elements of low atomic weight are combined even *with an infinitesimal weight* of radiations of an element of high atomic weight, and these neutrons in turn readily combine with other elements with which they come in contact ; and while these elements of the third state do not necessarily become changed, they become unstable and again subject to further changes. Millikan quotes the case of " a bit of beryllium mixed with an infinitesimal amount of radium emanation . . ." where one of the neutrons released enters the nucleus of an atom of silver and thus raises the atomic weight of the silver one unit, the silver becoming extra heavy, still retaining its chemical properties, but becoming unstable and proceeding to throw out a negative electron and transforming itself into cadmium. To be sure, these changes were the result of experimental procedures, but we cannot be assured that any combination of elements might not produce just as profound changes, either constructive or destructive. This would be particularly true when we consider the methods we employ to release the inherent energy in seemingly inert substance. If our methods are sufficient to release energy we cannot be assured that they might not be transmuted.

A further problem in potentization presents itself to our inquiring minds. If our methods are sufficiently practical to release these energies (and we must admit that the potential powers of our high potencies often startle us with their reaction) we may well inquire to just what degree the atoms of the elements are broken up in these substances. Unquestionably there is some definite ratio of energy release from the various elements, but to what extent trituration or succussion touches the atomic structure itself we do not know. If we could know that our application of force to these substances actually broke up the atom, we would recognize as a corollary that the destruction of the elemental atom and the consequent release of protons and neutrons tended toward the actual formation of different elements, with different atomic structures, and that these in turn had their own rates of energy which might be stabilized or unstabilized under certain conditions and combinations.

This suggests further study of the composite substances, such as the plant remedies. It has not yet been demonstrated that living substance contains radioactive elements, but when we consider the implication of such experiments as those cited by Millikan we may question the reaction set up by breaking down elements of various atomic weights even in the lower registers and their interaction. Further, the reaction of these changing energies upon the molecular construction of the individual is something upon which we may ponder.

Seemingly, these problems are beyond the scope of the physician. We feel impelled to know some of our materia medica and a few simple principles for the administration of our remedies. In other words, we naturally take a near-sighted view of our work. If we take the wider view—the phenomenological view—we see that these problems demand a more thorough understanding of our work ; they express only a proper appreciation of our science and art.

Even the United States Department of Public Health is recognizing the fact that where selenium is found near the surface—which occurs in only a few places in this country— the impaired health of the community makes continued habitation impractical and dangerous. Selenium ranks 34 in the scale of atomic weights, between arsenic and bromine, and falls considerably below those radioactive elements that have long been known to be dangerous neighbours.

The series of aeroplane accidents on our Pacific Coast in 1936-7 has been attributed to the influence of uranium fields where the deposits approach the surface in certain places in California. Uranium is one of our very heaviest elements, number 92 in the scale ; it is highly radioactive, and it is believed that these radiations disturbed the delicate instruments so they were useless, hence the tragedies occurred.

Consider the patient with a heart condition, who cannot endure high altitudes. We recognize this important modality, and look for the profound reason behind it. We are told that cosmic rays are five and one-half times as destructive at an altitude of 14,000 feet as at sea level. Cosmic rays are essentially destructive to all elements, especially the radio-active. Subjecting a patient hampered through his circulatory system, his vital balance already impaired, to forces known to be destructive might easily be fatal. It may be significant that these heart conditions often fall into the class of those conditions we recognize as being syphilitic or sycotic in origin (using *syphilitic* and *sycotic* in the sense of either the acquired disease or the inherited dyscrasia). The remedies applicable in these conditions, as we have pointed out previously, are remedies that in the majority are rated in the radioactive group.

On the other hand, the patient who suffers from atmospheric pressure and the dampness of sea level flourishes at higher altitudes. We have previously discussed the problem of sycosis as a probable over-stimulation of growth and development of certain body cells. If this individual is exposed to increased bombardment by the cosmic rays, this tends to balance the diseased state, and the patient enjoys a more stable equilibrium.

Here in the field of the atom lies the final answer to our questions of sickness and health—the problems of conception, growth, vital balance, decay. Here lies the answer to our problem of cure—maintenance of normal development, retention of vital balance, insurance against premature decay. This is a challenge to the scientist with an understanding of the homœopathic principles and their application, or to the homœopathic scientist who comprehends the phenomena of the structure of the universe. Not in a study of the individual sick cells, but of the universe and universal law, reflected in the universal structure of each elemental atom, shall we find our clarified view.

CHAPTER XXXIV

THE DEFLECTED CURRENT

WE are told that light waves travel in a certain direction until they meet some obstacle, when they are deflected at an angle proportionate to the angle of interference. We are told that our remedies are curative in conditions closely similar to those produced by the remedy in a healthy human being. The science of optics can give us, with a very small percentage of error, the measurement of the light waves, their angles of deflection and the measurements necessary to correct vision or to utilize the light waves in some practical manner. In other words, there is a definite measurable approach through known laws to the application of light waves to our modern needs ; and we may be assured that with a growth in our needs, and a greater understanding of those laws and measurements, future generations will be able to utilize light waves to a far greater degree than is thought of at the present time.

The homœopathic laws are fundamental ; we understand many of them ; we utilize them. Unfortunately, we have no such instruments of precision by which we can measure the obstacles to the curative waves of our remedies. Therefore we have no uniform results from our remedies such as we might expect from the vast armamentarium of remedies and the compilation of knowledge and experience garnered by successful homœopathic students since the time of Hahnemann.

Some of our confreres will say, at this point, that such instruments of precision are being used by homœopathic physicians at the present time ; that they are daily being perfected and that the results are increasingly satisfactory. No doubt all of this is true ; yet for the average homœopathic student we feel that such means are not yet available, or if available, the technique has not been sufficiently mastered by the average physician to be handled with accuracy ; or perhaps the degree of perfection (or imperfection) of such instruments interferes with capable usage.

However this may be, our thesis has to do with the average homœopathic physician, and may be reduced to that all too well known question : Why are our results not uniformly satisfactory ? *Why doesn't the seemingly indicated remedy always work ?*

Of course there are the answers known to every physician of whatever school, and some that only the homœopathic physician recognizes.

One obvious reason is the pathological condition of the patient. The röentgenologist and the surgeon are more apt to know about such pathological obstacles than is the homœopathic physician, but they so lack the means to cure that their knowledge teaches them only to remove offending tissue ; perhaps the patient recovers by the aid of beneficent nature. It is trite but true that more mistakes are made by not looking than by not knowing.

On the other hand, there are serious homœopathic students who have come to believe that treatment of patho-logical conditions by X-ray or radium dissipates, rather than cures, the pathological tissue. Certainly we have seen the results of over-exposure to such treatments, with the insuperable obstacle to cure that has been thus raised. Destruction of normal tissue, under such treatment, may prove as dangerous to the patient's health as lack of treat-ment ; and the relation of metastases to surgery, X-ray or radium treatment is still an open question in the minds of many close observers.

Then there are the states which arise from mechanical obstruction, non-pathological but the actual presence of a foreign body, which gives rise to reflex symptoms of exceed-ingly troublesome nature. Of course the remedy does not and cannot cure such symptoms so long as the causative factor remains. Persistent earaches or coryzas in children who have inserted small objects into the ear or nose have their counterpart in the suffering of adults, often from unusual minor accidents.

Psychic trauma, emotional stresses of varying degrees and

insistence, are factors that we, as homœopathic prescribers, should understand and weigh thoroughly in view of the patient's symptomatology. However, frequently the patient does not consider his private affairs the business of any outsider, even of the physician, and keeps these important items to himself. Or he may be so used to bearing his own burdens that he does not recognize them as having any weight in the case ; or he may (consciously or unconsciously) distort the picture of his own mental stress so much that even if he reveals the difficulty under which he is labouring, the whole picture may be of little help to the physician in analysing the case.

It was Hahnemann himself who emphasized the fact that nothing was so deleterious to health as unhappy domestic conditions ; that these conditions could, and often did, prove insuperable obstacles to cure. It is fortunate that th٠ *simillimum* often can take the additional tension from the patient, or may lift off one series of symptoms ; but so long as these strains persist under the surface, one cannot expect cure. Nevertheless, if the physician does not realize that these underlying influences exist, he may fall so far short of helping the patient that he may imperil his own belief in the homœopathic possibilities of cure, as well as the confidence of the patient.

Over-anxiety, worry, constant financial stress, the tension of maintaining speed in one's work, peculiar industrial demands—all these and many like stresses have developed unusual influences upon our patients during the past few years, and have correspondingly lowered the percentage of possible cures. They have served to deflect the current of cure in whole or in part ; and the homœopathic system of medicine is not at fault in such deflection of cure so long as these conditions remain a vital part of the patient's life.

Along with such conditions the physician has to fight the increasing use of sedatives, bromides, narcotics, analgesics— all forms of drugging which offer the patient some retreat from the pressure of the modern age or some measure of relief from pain, either mental or physical. Often the physician does not know of the home prescribing of the patient with such products of the pharmacist, but modern advertising keeps these products before the mind of the public to such an extent that they have proved one of the greatest barriers to cure ever known.

In these cases one must know the obstacle to cure if he is to be able to serve the patient with any degree of real assistance ; although it is one of the greatest boons of homœopathy that so many of our remedies have in themselves the power to antidote massive drugs, and so release the vital power inherent in the patient himself, with the corresponding response toward cure.

Cosmetics may prove the obstacle to cure just as surely as narcotics or coal-tar derivatives. Many cosmetic preparations contain substances advertised to suppress perspiration, eruptions, or to remove hair growth. Most physicians see cases definitely traceable to such measures. The suppressed eruptions and their sequelae are endless. We have seen a case of progressive paralysis in a young woman which she herself traced to the use of a depilatory preparation.

An eminent contemporary prescriber reported a case of a persistent *Coccus cacti* cough which refused to yield—until he ordered the young woman to stop the use of her lipstick, when the cough ceased.

Even the " old school " pharmaceutical journals are beginning to report a great variety of cases which have been traced to perfumes or perfumed cosmetics, and even to cite the physiological action of their ingredients. It is notable that some of these cases occurred, not in users of the cosmetic products, but in those associated with them. The homœopathic physician understands the power of ambergris, musk, etc., to produce symptoms in the potency. Hahnemann taught the power of olfaction on sensitive patients. Modern medical lore is full of the allergic reactions of sensitive patients to a variety of substances, in the most minute form. When even the dominant school of medicine recognizes this hazard, the homœopathic physician must never neglect consideration of such a deflection of the current.

Then there is the problem of diet. The so-called soft drinks follow closely the record of home drugging in distorting the case. The modern craze for slender figures, with the unbalanced diets prescribed by the laity, may be an obstacle to cure ; not because the physician cannot correct the condition with a proper balanced diet plus an indicated remedy, but because of the psychological barrier—the unwillingness to accept a suitable diet with the corresponding normal weight. In other words, the patient who suffers willingly from malnutrition can be brought back to normal only if his co-operation is gained, or if the case comes to the physician before dangerous physiological changes set in. On the other hand, there is the malnutrition resulting from an unbalanced diet directly traceable to depressed budget ; this condition has grown rapidly during the depression years and the effects are still shown in many cases. This has to be met not only with the homœopathic remedy but with economic equilibrium and a well thought out diet if the patient is to be cured. Here we meet an economic obstacle that is often beyond the help of the physician.

The question of proper exercise would seem to lie within the province of the physician. We recall one case, however, where the patient, a woman past middle life, was instructed to get out of the house, into the open, and cultivate her interest in wild flowers, thus getting her interests outside herself along with fresh air and sunshine. We supposed the prescription was being filled, as we were greeted with fresh wild flowers every call we made, but she did not seem to gain in strength nor did her colour improve. Some time later (after she left us for a more sympathetic physician) we found that her husband faithfully went to the fields and gathered fresh flowers for the vases, while she rested from the prospect of his endeavours in her behalf.

There are patients who cannot take strenuous exercise because of pathological obstacles. There are patients who are so restricted by circumstances that they get little opportunity for exercise in the open air. But such patients are usually chronics with a long history and a poor prognosis ; we usually accept the situation and do the best we can toward homœopathic palliation, and surprising as it may be to us, we sometimes approach cure in spite of the difficulties. But the patient who can co-operate, but will not, and perhaps even leads us to believe she has made the attempt, herself deflects the current of cure at its very source. Then we

18

question the value of our prescription and wonder why the indicated remedy failed to work.

One of our hardest problems is the patient who cannot seem to rally—the old chronic, with a long but seemingly not overwhelming history, and with a clear picture of a remedy. Somewhere here there is an obstacle to cure and we must plumb the history—physical, mental, emotional—to remove that obstacle or measure it, and to me sure as well our remedy and its potency, to determine whether it is the *simillimum* in likeness of symptomatology and energy.

Another obstacle to cure is the ease with which the physician's judgment may be overbalanced in favour of the patient's favourite symptom. This may seem a trifling matter, but frequent repetition of a troublesome symptom may so warp the true picture of the case that the symptomatology seems to reflect an entirely different remedy than those true, but less conspicuous indications, that are actually present. The patient does this unconsciously by remembering the most troublesome factors and forgetting the seemingly minor items that should furnish the clue to the remedy.

We have discussed some of the obstacles to cure as they affect the patient or the physician. Let us discuss the other side of the problem : the remedy.

Here our first problem is the source of the remedy itself. How close to Hahnemann's standard did the source of our remedy approach ? In other words, how carefully did the homœopathic pharmacist identify the source of his supply ? Is the plant identical with the botanical source of our proving ? We cannot expect a *Rhus tox.* case, for instance, to be cured with some other member of the family, if we have depended upon the proving of *Rhus tox.* as our guide. Here we enter the field of similars instead of the *simillimum*. Was the original supply fresh and in good condition ? Substances of inferior quality cannot provide a good potency. With what degree of thoroughness did the pharmacist follow Hahnemann's instructions for potentization ? With what degree of thoroughness did the provers follow instructions ?

We must be able to depend absolutely upon the sources of our remedies, and if there has been carelessness in gathering the original substance, in any part of the process of making the potency, in contamination in handling the potency or in discrepancies in recording the provings, then we cannot but expect that the current of cure will be deflected. All these details are known to the homœopathic prescriber, but we cannot refrain from pointing out that these details may spell the difference between life and death, certainly between cure and failure, in many of our cases where there seems to be no reason to expect a deflection of the current of cure.

We question whether the provings were made under proper control. How many entered into the proving? How accurately was the substance, the origin of the potency, labelled? Inaccurate labelling might be the difference in possible cure or deflection by an insurmountable obstacle.

Weighing the symptoms of the patient against those of the remedy is one of our major problems ; but an even more important problem is the weighing of symptoms of the proving itself. How great a value, we ask ourselves, shall we place upon those symptoms occasionally or rarely produced in a proving? We are told, for instance, that the time aggravation which is almost a keynote of *Kali carb.* appeared in only one prover, yet it has been clinically confirmed so frequently that we often think of it as one of the leading symptoms of *Kali carb.*—or when we think of the 3 a.m. aggravation we immediately think of *Kali carb.*, in spite of the fact that Kent's *Repertory* lists a number of remedies with this modality.

It is important that we use every means within our power to determine whether or not the occasional symptom comes from the individuality of the remedy or whether it is a deflection of the remedy's dynamis through idiosyncrasies of the patient or through something the patient may do or may use that distorts the reaction. Here is a patient, for instance, who cannot take *Hepar sulph.* without producing a symptom not appearing in any of our *Hepar* provings—a sensation as if a finger and thumb were pressing either side of the larynx. Is this a valuable symptom or is it an individual reaction of no value?

Hahnemann gave us very clear directions for making provings, and instructed us that in every case the usual habits and diet of the prover remain at ordinary level during the proving, so that we might knqw whether or not the symptoms were produced by the remedy or by changes in the prover's habits. However, it is conceivable that such things as diet, etc., even if the patient had become accustomed to them, might deflect the current of symptoms in like degree to the disturbing element in the dietary. We reflect that such articles of diet as coffee, which we are taught affects the action of certain remedies when prescribed for curative purposes, might in like degree modify the reaction of the remedy in its proving, either to completely nullify part of the symptomatology or to modify it to an entirely different picture. Thus we must use every care in adopting casual provings. In the case of Hahnemann's provings, he reduced them to what approaches a mathematical formula. He carefully weighed the habits, diet and general state of health as manifested by symptomatic reaction of each prover before such prover was accepted for service. This data was subtracted, as it were, from such symptomatology as appeared during the course of the proving or within reasonable time thereafter, and the remaining symptoms were credited to the remedy action. Moreover, this procedure was well controlled by the number o: provers for each remedy. These details were watched witl the precision characteristic of Hahnemann.

A word about keynotes as a possible obstacle to cure i not out of place. Keynote symptoms have proved them selves as of almost equal degree a bane or a blessing. With our vast array of remedies the average homœopathic physician learns well the polychrests ; thereafter, depending upon their relationship to his practice, he tends to depenc upon memorizing a more or less brief outline of remedies Many remedies he knows only by keynotes. If these key-notes are used as a reference to materia medica study they serve well, but they are very dangerous for a basis in prescribing. If he prescribes solely on the keynote he may, and often does, remove the conspicuous symptoms ; but this may serve only as an obstacle to cure by deflecting the current of symptomatology and thus distorting the picture of the patient himself.

" The physician should distinctly understand the following conditions ; what is curable·in diseases in general, and in each individual case in particular. . . . He should clearly comprehend what is curative in drugs in general, and in each drug in particular. . . . He should be governed by distinct reasons, in order to insure recovery, by adapting what is curative in medicines to what he has recognized as undoubtedly morbid in a patient. . . . Finally, when the physician knows in each case the obstacles in the way of recovery, and how to remove them, he is prepared to act thoroughly, and to the purpose, as a true master of the art of healing."

Chapter XXXV

MODERN MEDICATION AND THE HOMŒOPATHIC PRINCIPLES

LIKE all principles, those of homœopathy have been discovered and evolved through the crucibles of time, experimentation, and increasing enlightenment. Like all principles, too, they stand whether or not they have the ascription of those who profess to be their adherents. They are principles that, to those who understand and seek to apply them and to those who benefit from their application, stand pre-eminent, unchangeable, in spite of all changes in therapeutic fashions. To principles there is no time element. Natural law knows no ancient, no modern. Time offers only the greater opportunity for examination of the results of applied principles, the action of the natural laws ; and evolution knows not the meaning of fashion.

The word *modern* must always be used in a comparative sense. This is never appreciated more keenly than when considered in the light of medical practice, and those elements of the practice of to-day that have survived the crucible of time have rightly become recognized as the principles of the art.

Medicine, while always dealing with the ills of mankind, has passed through a continuous barrage of " modern " discoveries. Greater possibilities of investigation of the functions of the body have increased our knowledge of life processes and the circumstances of living ; and this increase in knowledge has been of inestimable value in dealing with human suffering. But therapeutics, as demonstrated by modern medicine, is still in a state similar to that of the past, in that the discovery or development of the day is the seeming answer to almost all therapeutic problems. This is another way of saying that in spite of the increased knowledge of the mechanism of the body, no guiding principles have been discovered by the dominant school of medicine that are sure and certain indications in the field of therapeutics. That means there is no test but that of experience for any therapeutic agent, and modern medicine, despite the period of its discovery, still finds itself on a basis of empiricism rather than of true science.

Consider the discovery of the synthetic group of drugs. There has been a continuous procession of these substances over a period of years. Aspirin, luminol, the phenols, the sulphanilamides, the vitamins and numerous others. Each discovery has been hailed as a modern development of science for the conquering or alleviation of the ills of mankind. Sober investigation of the claims of these therapeutic measures astounds us with the conviction that in almost every instance the target at which these measures are aimed is a single symptom or, at most, a small group of symptoms, and not at the patient himself. In most cases the discovery of such a therapeutic agent has been met with loud acclaim and ardent advertising ; its use became widespread very shortly. Soon the sincere students of science perceived, through their laboratory research and from clinical observations, that there was another face to the seeming curative action of the substance, that was not without danger to the patient ; and therefore warnings were sent out that there should not be too free use of the substances except under the most careful observation. In the meantime the fashion of use had spread, especially among those who always seek the easy road in therapeutics, the uninstructed and those who are addicted to self-dosing, with a corresponding amount of further damage to health.

Such an agent was aspirin. First advanced for its harmless sedative properties in the control of pain, it was widely used and in considerable amounts, by physician and laymen alike, until its depressant properties came to be respected by careful therapeutists. The American Medical Association found it advisable to publish warnings against the use of this substance which was commonly sold under the trade name of aspirin ; but the use of the substance was not curtailed to any marked degree except by the most careful prescribers. It had become a cure-all for domestic use and all too often in hospitals and by physicians who sought first the suppression of the distressing symptoms rather than the cure of the patient.

Homœopathic physicians have long known the dangers of suppressive measures, and have always had due respect for the innate powers of any medicament. It was Hahnemann who observed that any drug was poisonous if dangerous dosage were given. Therefore it is to be expected that homœopathic physicians early recognized the dangers of the synthetic drugs, among them the coal-tar derivatives. The ability of the trained homœopath to observe and correlate symptoms made it a foregone conclusion that he would easily trace the depressed vitality, the heart attacks, and many collapsed conditions, to the frequent use of aspirin and like pain-killers.

The homœopathic physician is likewise trained to realize the dangers of suppressed or masked symptoms ; that pain has its beneficent aspect as a guidepost, and that the discomforts of an acute cold or grippe cannot be suppressed without grave danger to the ultimate health of the patient. The prevalence of the symptom, " never been well since ", is proof of this.

The phenols, and especially phenobarbital, were hailed loudly as curative, and especially as palliative of many ills. It was not long before their deadly nature was discovered, and the warnings were posted against their use. They are still used extensively, but much more conservatively than formerly. In many of these instances, it is the early dangerous action that is discovered and the later, more insidious and long lasting effects are undiscovered or ignored until too late ; these become constitutional and therefore are unrecognized.

Of course all these effects, from first to last, are homœopathic proof of the potentialities of cure that lie in these synthetic drugs. To the homœopath, however, there should be but one criterion for their use—the similarity of symptoms produced in the healthy for application to like ills in the sick.

The popular sulphanilamides are one of the best instances of the powers and dangers of synthetic drugs. They have been hailed for their powerful action in infections of many—one is tempted to say all—kinds. It is true that in laboratory and clinic they have proven this power. But along with the proven power of destroying invading organisms they have a like danger to normal cell balance ; this has been recognized by those who developed the drug to the point where careful therapeutists will not use these agents without keeping careful laboratory check on the blood stream and other functions of the patient.

Probably more variations of this group of drugs have been developed than of any other that has become popular. When sulphanilamide was first publicly recognized and marketed, it was permitted to fall into the hands of laymen who had read glowing accounts of its value and who decided that they could cure themselves of all their ailments with this wonderful panacea. Numbers of these hopeful sufferers purchased, and many deaths resulted. Manufacturers of the products were obliged to keep a closer watch on the production and distribution, and research chemists set about developing less dangerous combinations.

The fact remains that where medicinal agents are capable of eradicating organisms by any other method than by stimulation of the dynamic force to the point where nature itself balances the scale, there is danger to the patient, sooner or later.

It is no doubt true that sulphanilamide and its variations have a comparatively good record in such conditions as pneumonia and like infections. That is, a good record compared to that of the dominant school where pneumonia is a dangerous and often fatal disease. The sulphonamides have so far given a more creditable record than the serum treatments of pneumonia which were so well sung only a few years ago ; and in the use of the sulphonamides only prompt use is necessary—one may omit the typing and thus save time. In fact, it has been said by eminent authorities on the use of the sulphonamides that in infections they must be used promptly in the onset of the infection of whatever kind, or they are useless.

Let us analyse this situation. Here we are given a therapeutic agent that will kill the invading organism, with a corresponding dangerous action against normal functions of the body ; yet potent as this is, it is of no value against the invading organism after that has become established. Are we to believe that its danger to the normal cells of the patient has diminished in proportion to its possibilities of help against the invader ?

It has been many years since the possibility of sterile death has been acknowledged—the blood stream being sterilized of invading organisms, yet death results. This is as true now as then ; and the danger may be imminent or retarded in relation to the amount of the crude dosage or the frequency of its administration. Careful observers in both schools of medicine have noted the slow return to normal health of patients " cured ", i.e. the acute infection having been overcome, by heroic methods—or as we may better say, by the application of forces outside the normal functions of the body. Therefore, although the invading organisms have been limited in action, the system has to overcome the effects of the infection plus the toxic effects of the treatment.

Now let us consider the sulphonamides in relation to the homœopathic principles. We might consider, in the light of our thesis, any or all of the synthetic drugs, but so far as we know there has been no effort to exhibit the potential powers of the substances through the well-known and thoroughly tried method of Hahnemann—that of proving the remedy on the healthy human being. Such an attempt has been made in the case of sulphanilamide, notably by Dr. Allan D. Sutherland ; the results of this fragmentary proving were published in the *Homœopathic Recorder* for September 1940.

Dr. Sutherland's conclusions were that this substance, potentized, has great possibilities as a homœopathic remedy when we have more clearly demonstrated its field of usefulness by the sure guide of the symptomatic outlines that our principles demand ; these are the only guides which provide safety in cure rather than uncertain palliation of a condition that the patient later has to overcome through his natural vitality, or else succumb to in some other and more deeply constitutional form at a later date.

The homœopathic adage that we try to cure the patient rather than the disease might well be supplemented by the statement that we do not presume to snatch the patient from an acute illness from which, by the grace of his dynamic energies, he might well recover (acute illnesses being always self-limiting) to foist upon him a constitutional condition plus the imposed drug illness, from which he may never recover.

The results of the homœopathic remedies in such infections as pneumonia, grippe, streptococcus, staphylococcus and other generalized or local infections have been more remarkable than in any other system of medication. This is a simple way of saying that the natural laws, upon which homœopathy is founded and upon which our principles are based, work just as surely in serious, swift-paced onslaughts of disease as in any other condition. It is true that in some of these conditions the system is more deeply involved and death more imminent than in many conditions we are called upon to treat. It is also true that many of these serious infections were cured before the laboratories were at hand to furnish accurate diagnoses, and that very often the most prominent result of a laboratory diagnosis is to weaken the courage of the physician, the patient, and the patient's family.

The homœopathic physician recognizes another important principle in these serious states : the more acute the case, the more the infection strikes at the life of the patient, the more clearly indicative are the symptoms. Obscuration of symptoms (unless produced by crude drugging) is very rare in a case of acute infection. The homœopathic remedy works regardless of the name of the disease, and works, moreover, toward a true and complete cure, without sequelæ or constitutional involvement.

The value of vitamins in the diet has been a burning subject among research chemists and therapeutists alike. The source of vitamins in natural foods, especially raw fruits, has been recognized for some time ; and of course sources of synthetic vitamins have been discovered and their use urged through the drug houses. One simple but obvious fact seems always to be overlooked by the manufacturing chemists—that while chemically the synthetic product may vary little from the natural, there is a difference which is recognizable in results, sometimes far removed in time from the experimental stage. It is hardly likely that a patient would suffer from too many vitamins through a normal diet ; the vitamin is normally balanced with the other food values.

With the increased regard for vitamins as a necessity of life, we are now under a barrage of foodstuffs where added synthetic vitamins are an ineradicable part of the diet. Since it has been found that these substances are necessary to life and development, argue the laboratory chemists, therefore as a nation we must take advantage of this source of increased energy and vigour ; and since the synthetic vitamins have the same chemical construction and are easily available at a comparatively low cost, we must use these vitamins to the fullest extent, therefore they are introduced into many basic foods such as flour, etc. Thus we have a business venture which is very profitable to the producers of the vitamins, and it becomes almost impossible for an individual to escape a diet heavily laden with synthetic vitamins.

Now, however, the careful research men who investigate carefully all sides of the question and take time to correlate facts, are beginning to voice the conclusion that after long and critical study they find there is as great danger from too many vitamins as from too few, and perhaps more. This is a statement in accord with homœopathic principles, and with the laws of nature governing balance in all things : " The amount necessary to effect any change in nature is the least possible " ; " Action and reaction are equal and opposite."

The manufacturing chemist states in his literature that it has been determined that the normal vitamin requirement is from 3 to 25 milligrams per day. We may expect that overdosing with vitamins, which have a constructive and maintenance value, would have two definite reactions : first, a destructive action proportionate to its normal constructive action ; and second, the permanent disability of the system to react to normal vitamin intake. This latter is comparable to the effect of insulin administration in the diabetic patient ; he soon loses his ability to produce the necessary secretion in his own economy. This is another illustration of the loss of a function by the need being supplied through no effort of the patient, and evolution bears witness to the fact that what a creature does not use he must lose. Thus the excess supply of vitamins robs the body of its normal reception of the natural vitamins.

One can hardly conceive of the effect of a high vitamin intake on the younger generation in the light of this conclusion. And we can hardly fail to consider the results of the unrestricted administration of these elements in future generations : will they be able to assimilate them from natural sources, or will there be, after a time, some radical change in the human economy to compensate ?

In particular, we may inquire regarding the reactions in the special functions : will these functions be permanently affected ? For instance, it has been demonstrated that vitamins C and D help to overcome rickets, and that a certain amount of these are necessary for the proper growth and development of the bony structure. It has also been demonstrated that excessive doses will cause rickets. Since vitamin E is supposed to stimulate the generative function, will massive dosing destroy or impair this function ? We might continue this analogy through the list of vitamins so far isolated and studied.

It is well for us, as homœopathic physicians, not to overlook the potentialities of the synthetics in the field of therapeutics ; but we must examine them carefully in the light of our well-proven homœopathic principles, remembering also that the findings of the clinic do not necessarily bear the same relationship to the human patient as to the laboratory animal, and that the secondary results may vary widely from—nay, be directly opposite to—the primary results which appear to be so brilliant and satisfactory.

We must remember that our homœopathic laws, if they are natural laws, as we have every reason to believe, are still worthy of our consideration and that no sure guidance has yet been found that is not in accordance with those laws ; and that the test of time must be applied in every instance of a new discovery that has not been tried according to known law. It is foolish to reject the new just because it is new, but it is even more foolish to accept every new finding blindly without fully testing its validity when we have at hand all the means for sound procedure, means which the dominant school so far has failed to accept.